Your Baby's Sleep in the First Year

Excerpt from *The Science of Mother-Infant Sleep*

Edited by Wendy Middlemiss, PhD &
Kathleen Kendall-Tackett, PhD, IBCLC, FAPA

Praeclarus Press, LLC

www.PraeclarusPress.com

Praeclarus Press, LLC

2504 Sweetgum Lane

Amarillo, Texas 79124 USA

806-367-9950

www.PraeclarusPress.com

DISCLAIMER
The information contained in this publication is advisory only and is not intended to replace sound clinical judgment or individualized patient care. The author disclaims all warranties, whether expressed or implied, including any warranty as the quality, accuracy, safety, or suitability of this information for any particular purpose.

ISBN 978-1-939807-58-8

Cover Design: Ken Tackett
Acquisition & Development: Kathleen Kendall-Tackett
Copy Editing: Chris Tackett
Layout & Design: Nelly Murariu
Operations: Scott Sherwood

Table of Contents

1

Is Your Baby's Sleep a Problem? Or Is It Just Normal?

Tracy Cassels, Sarah Ockwell-Smith,
Wendy Middlemiss, Kathleen Kendall-Tackett
Helen Stevens, & Darcia Narvaez

Most new parents complain about lack of sleep. Many are also concerned that their babies have a "sleep problem," and that what they are experiencing isn't "normal." So they search books, ask friends and family—or even their doctor—what they should do about their child's problematic sleep patterns. And they worry about it—a lot.

Part of this epidemic of parental angst about children's sleep is that we live in a culture in which parents are repeatedly told that they *need* to worry about their child's sleep, that there will be dire consequences if their child doesn't get enough sleep. Another problem is that most new parents, having had little experience with children prior to having their own, have little awareness about what truly is "normal" when it comes to infant sleep.

Simply being made aware of normal sleep patterns can help alleviate the stress and anxiety parents feel, leading to happier times for the entire family.

So What Is Normal?

This chapter describes some of the more common sleep concerns parents have with the hope that they can see them as normal, developmental stages for their child.

The Critical Roles of Feeding Method and Changes in Development

"My child wakes every hour, all day and night, to feed."

Whether it's every hour, or every two hours, or even three, parents are often concerned when their young infant is waking regularly for feedings. This concern is not surprising given the focus on "sleeping through the night" that our culture pushes. But sleeping through the night is not biologically normal, especially for a breastfeeding baby.

At the time of birth, a baby's stomach can only hold a teaspoonful worth of milk, meaning that he or she will need to feed frequently to meet the many demands for energy that accompany this period of growth. Although the stomach grows relatively quickly, the fat and protein content in human breast milk is much lower than in the milk of other mammals, and thus infants are required to feed often, resulting in greater night wakings (Ball, 2003; 2009).

Human milk, being designed for infants who need to feed on cue day *and* night, is easily and quickly digested. Formula, however, is typically made from the milk of another species–cows–and is higher in fat while also containing myriad additives that make it more difficult, and thus slower, to digest. This can affect infant sleep, resulting in unnaturally deeper infant sleep (more time spent in stage 3-4; Butte, Jensen, Moon, Glaze, & Frost Jr., 1992). Stage 3-4 is most difficult to arouse from to terminate breathing pauses. This is especially true for infants who are arousal deficient. Longer stages of Stage 3-4 sleep could potentially diminish the infant's capacity to maintain sufficient oxygen. Even so, formula use does not necessarily provide parents with more sleep overall (Doan, Gardiner, Gay, & Lee, 2007; Kendall-Tackett, Cong, & Hale, 2011).

Infants whose primary source of energy is breast milk will often wake frequently to nurse, something that is essential for the breastfeeding relationship to continue (Ball, 2009). However, regardless of feeding status, many infants wake regularly during the night (Weinraub, Bender, Friedman, Susman, Knoke, Bradley, et al., 2012). *Waking through the night is normal and biologically adaptive.* In fact, though it is often reported that sleep patterns consolidate in the second year, the pattern differs in breastfed children.

Breastfeeding mothers may wake more often, but report greater total sleep time. For example, in a study of 6,410 mothers of infants 0 to 12 months old, exclusively breastfeeding mothers reported both more wakings and more total sleep time compared with mixed- or exclusively formula-feeding mothers (Kendall-Tackett, Cong, & Hale, 2011). The exclusively breastfeeding mothers reported less daytime fatigue, more energy, less anger and irritability, and lower levels of depressive symptoms.

Interestingly, mothers who were both breast and formula-feeding reported fewer hours of sleep than exclusively breastfeeding mothers, *and there was no significant difference between the mixed- and formula-feeding mothers on any of the outcome measures* (Kendall-Tackett, Cong, & Hale, 2011). This is important because new mothers are often pushed to supplement to "get more rest." These results, consistent with the findings of Doan et al. (2007), suggest that *supplementing actually results in less sleep—not more.*

Night wakings continue to be common as breast-feeding infants mature. In a study of children who were breastfeeding at age 2, night wakings were common throughout the second year of life. This pattern of night wakings is commonly observed in cultures where co-sleeping and full-term (aka, "extended") breastfeeding are more common (Elias, Nicolson, Bora, & Johnston, 1986).

Night Wakings Protect Infants

Night wakings have been reported as being more common in infants who bedshare with a parent, yet the wakings and bedsharing (when done safely) may actually protect infants from SIDS (Mosko, Richard, & McKenna, 1997; Mosko, Richard, McKenna, & Drummond, 1996). The critical period for SIDS is up to 8 months of age (with the peak at 2 to 3 months), and night wakings may serve as a protective mech-anism. In fact, if we look at parenting historically and cross-culturally, frequent night wakings, coupled with co-sleeping and breastfeeding, are the norm for which we should be comparing other infant sleep behaviors.

"My child was sleeping through the night and suddenly stopped."

Imagine you've been waking regularly with night feeds and arousals, but as time passes they are decreasing. Then you realize you're now sleeping in nice, long chunks. Hours of sleep all at once! And it's wonderful. Then suddenly, as quickly as it came, it's gone. Your wonderful, sleeping-through-the-night child is suddenly waking again. This experience, which is a reality for many, can cause frustration and despair accompanied by the feeling that you've done something wrong, or that you must do something to get their uninterrupted sleep back again.

Here's the thing: You didn't *do* anything. *A return to night waking after periods of sleeping through the night is entirely normal.* Many children's sleep will cycle like this for a while. In fact, researchers looking at sleep patterns have found that often between 6 and 12 months, infants who had previously been sleeping long stretches suddenly start to wake more frequently at night (Scher, 1991, 2001). In one long-term study looking at child sleep between three and 42 months found that there was *no* stability in night wakings, or even sleep duration, during this time (Scher, Epstein, & Tirosh, 2004).

What Causes the Change in Sleeping Pattern?

There are likely a variety of reasons, unique to each child. For some, it may be a growth spurt or teething. For others, it may be a cognitive leap that has them buzzing more so than usual, or the appearance of separation anxiety. Just recently a study reported that babies tend to wake more often when they are learning to crawl. And for some, we may never know the actual reason. But as children age, and each develops a circadian rhythm, they will go through cycles of sleep–some more convenient for parents than others.

Parents need to be aware that these changes are entirely normal, even though they can be frustrating. Hopefully, once you know that changes are to be expected, you can be better prepared, or at least not add anxiety to the sleep disruptions you are forced to deal with once again.

"My child wakes up at 2 a.m., and is up for one to two hours!"

One mother remembers very clearly the first time her daughter ended up doing this. At around 14 months, she woke up in the middle of the night and didn't seem ready or able to go back to sleep for one to two hours no matter what strategies her parents tried. This continued regularly for a couple of months. And then as quickly as it started, it stopped, and hasn't happened again in over a year.

The "why" of this is relatively unknown—although researchers are continuing to explore the physiological underlyings of sleep—but we do know that extended night wakings like these are experienced by many children until around 3 years of age (Weinraub, Bender, Friedman, Susman, Knoke, Bradley et al., 2012). *Many times the wakings are brief and the child settles quickly. Other times settling takes longer. In either case, these wakings do not suggest your child has a sleep "problem."*

Increased night wakings, call-outs, and crying are more common around 6 months of age or so, and again as infants near 2 years of age. *These wakings may simply be one (of many) manifestations of separation anxiety experienced by the child*—a normal change resulting from infants learning that they exist separately from their caregivers (for a review, see Middlemiss, 2004).

Some argue that night wakings in toddlerhood are reflective of sleep problems, but these opinions are based on criteria that do not necessarily reflect the realities of infant sleep. Several studies found that night waking is relatively common between age 12 and 24 months (Richman, 1981; Goodlin-Jones, Burnham, Gaylor, & Anders 2001; Scher, 2000; Weinraub et al., 2013).

Thus, a parent's perceptions about what constitutes a sleep problem may be triggered by either a disconnect between expectations of uninterrupted sleep, and a toddler sleep pattern that arguably falls within the range of normal, or by the impact that night waking has on the parent's quality of sleep and daily functioning (Loutzenhiser, Ahlquist, & Hoffman 2012). However, although changes in sleep patterns may be inconvenient and frustrating, they are normal occurrences in the context of a healthy parent-child relationship.

When viewed as indicating problematic, rather than normal sleep patterns that will come and go, parents can experience greater stress and worry (Middlemiss, 2004). As we have learned from many parents, understanding that these night wakings are normal can go a long way toward making them more bearable.

The Importance of Understanding Individual Patterns in Sleep

"My child won't go to sleep before 10 p.m."

It is not uncommon in some parts of Western societies to assume that infants and young children must be in bed by, for example, 7 p.m. to develop "good sleep habits." *Unfortunately, that's just not the reality for many families, and it's not because parents are negligent in getting their infants to bed, but because some children simply have a different circadian rhythm, or a later schedule may work for the family.* Some children will continue this pattern into their toddler years and beyond.

Cross-cultural data on bedtimes for infants and toddlers shows that later bedtimes are actually quite frequent in predominantly Asian countries (Mindell, Sadeh, Wiegand, How, & Goh, 2010). Whereas the mean bedtime for children in predominantly Caucasian countries was found to be 8:42 p.m, it was a full hour later for predominantly Asian countries (with a mean at 9:44 p.m.), with the latest mean bedtime being 10:17 p.m. in Hong Kong. Notably, the rising time was also significantly later in these countries. A concurrent finding was that the vast majority of children in predominantly Asian countries sleep either in the parent's bed or room. *Thus, children who sleep with their parents may naturally have a sleep schedule closer to their parents owing to the sleeping arrangements.*

What is important to remember is that a late bedtime, in and of itself, is not a problem. If it poses a problem for the family as a whole, then parents may want to adjust the bedtime routine (Mindell, Telofski, Weigand, & Kurtz, 2009), or start the routine earlier in small increments in order to gradually move to an earlier bedtime (Richman, 1981).

"My child sleeps less than (or more than) the recommended amount no matter what I do!"

Most people have seen the "sleep guidelines" about how much sleep our children need at various stages. Parents are told that newborns should sleep around 16 to 18 hours, that at 2 years of age, children require a total of 13 hours sleep, and so on. *When researchers explore questions of how long infants and children should sleep, and what are healthy recommendations, the answers are not particularly clear,* and are often based on examining how much children *are sleeping* at different times in history (Matricciani, Olds, Blunden, Rigney, & Williams, 2012).

As parents, it is important to remember that these are *recommendations.* Each child is different, and the recommendations may not fit every child. Some will require much more sleep, and some will require less. *If a child is truly sleep deprived, there will be noticeable signs.* Signs of sleep deprivation include rubbing eyes, looking dazed, and not focusing on people or toys, becoming overly active late at night, and having a hard time waking up in the morning.

By paying attention to your child's cues and behaviors, you will be able to tell if your child is getting enough sleep, regardless of the exact number of hours he or she sleeps. Sleep is important, but there are many ways to get it apart from one long, uninterrupted stretch.[*]

Interestingly, researchers are now telling us that waking in the middle of the night is common in adulthood and was viewed as normal in past eras—the "first sleep" lasted about four hours, with an awake period in between, followed by a "second sleep" of another four hours (for more details, *At Day's Close: Night in Times Past* by Roger Ekirch: Norton, 2005).

Normal Parent Behaviors and Why They Won't Hurt Your Child

"My child is still sleeping in our bed."

Many parents who sleep with their child get comments along the lines of, "Your child will never leave if you don't move them" or "What about your sex life?" Parents end up questioning if they are doing the right thing for their children, or if they will end up with a 16-year-old who still wants to crawl into bed with mom and dad every night. First, let's address the question of when a child leaves the bed. Rest assured that your child will not be dragging you off to college so they can still sleep with you—*even if you don't force them out of the bed*.

The age at which children are ready to move into their own room varies widely, and bedsharing is quite common worldwide. Notably, bedsharing rates in

Scandinavian and Asian countries are much higher than those in the U.S. or Canada (Mindell, Sadeh, Wiegand, How, & Goh, 2010; Nelson & Taylor, 2001; Welles-Nystrom, 2005; for a review, see Cassels, 2013). Parents polled by one of the authors about the age at which their children initiated the move to another room report ages as young as 18 months, and as old as 10 years.

Some factors that influence the transition age include: having a sibling in the other room (thus being able to room-share with another child), the presence of a new baby in the bed (and needed attention to safety for the new baby and disrupted sleep for the older child), and the child's own developmental needs. Each family will need to consider the factors that are relevant for their particular child.

The research on extended bedsharing has not found any social, emotional, or cognitive detriment for bedsharing children relative to children who were placed in their own room in infancy (e.g., Abel, Park, Tipene-Leach, Finau, & Lennan, 2001; Barajas, Martin, Brooks-Gunn, & Hale, 2011; Keller & Goldberg, 2004; Okami, Weisner, & Olmstead, 2002).

The second issue that is often brought up has to do with the marital relationship when the family bed is utilized. New research looking at bedsharing and marital satisfaction has reported *no influence of bedsharing on the marital relationship when bedsharing is intentional* (Messmer, Miller, & Yu, 2012). When bedsharing is in reaction to child sleep problems, parents may report greater stress on their relationship, but it is likely that this is due to the problems associated with infant sleep problems. As to intimacy, parents of co-sleepers and bedsharers often find creative ways to make sure their needs are met as well. There are excellent (and humorous) blogs on the topic if you're in need of some extra assistance.

"My child only goes to sleep breastfeeding."

Most parents in the early months know how quickly an infant can go to sleep while breastfeeding. In fact, breastfeeding often is what sends our little ones to sleep. Although many people do not think twice about these behaviors when their infants are still quite tiny, they start to worry about it as the child ages. It doesn't help that "falling to sleep" while breastfeeding is listed as one of the sleep disorders by sleep researchers (Melzer & Mindell, 2006), and that often family and friends will tell you that you're harming your child, and that he or she will "never" learn to fall asleep on his or her own. Many "sleep experts" will recommend not letting your infant fall asleep on your breast for fear of creating this "bad habit" (Meltzer & Mindell, 2006), instead recommending that you rouse your little one before putting him or her down.

If you don't have a problem with breastfeeding your child until they are sleeping, and placing them down while sleeping, you don't need to worry about it for your child. How can we say this? First, a child who is tired enough will fall asleep with or without breastfeeding. Although falling asleep at the breast may remain a *preferred* way to fall asleep for a child (full of the closeness and intimacy that is so necessary for bonding), it will not be a necessary step.

As children age, they will fall asleep in various places and positions. *Young infants should not be forced to fall asleep without comfort; they may need to breastfeed to feel relaxed and safe enough to enter sleep.* Another factor to remember is that *all children eventually wean.* Breastfeeding and cuddling to sleep offer comfort for your child, a closeness that is associated with positive developmental outcomes. Children will seek this closeness as a natural part of development. This is not a bad thing; it is simply offering your child the closeness that is a natural part of growth and parenting.

If still uncertain, *be assured that breastfeeding is a natural way to help children sleep and provide important support for their growth.* Parents should know that breast milk in the evening contains more tryptophan (a sleep-inducing amino acid). Tryptophan is a precursor to serotonin, a vital hormone for brain function and development. In early life, tryptophan ingestion leads to more serotonin receptor development (Hibberd, Brooke, Carter, Haug, & Harzer, 1981).

Nighttime breast milk also has amino acids that promote serotonin synthesis (Delgado, 2006; Goldman, 1983; Lien, 2003). Serotonin makes the brain work better, keeps one in a good mood, and helps with sleep-wake cycles (Somer, 2009). So because of tryptophan and its wider effects, it *may be especially important for children to have evening or night breast milk for reasons beyond getting them to sleep.*

The other concern that is brought up is that infants and children who fall asleep at the breast (or even in-arms) often wake looking for the same environment in which they first fell asleep (Anders, Halpern, & Hua, 1992). This can lead to crying upon waking when they find themselves in a different environment, such as a crib.

For parents who bedshare and breastfeed, parents have reported decreased signaling as infants learn to seek mother's breast and latch themselves on to breastfeed when waking at night. *Though arousals continue to be greater in bedsharing dyads* (Mosko, Richard, & McKenna, 1997), *this natural interaction provides a soothing and simple way to care for infants as they wake.* In these cases, when the children are developmentally ready, putting them down nearly asleep, and letting them finish the process on their own, may help reduce wakings that result in signaling for the parent.

"My child only naps when I'm outside/walking/on me."

Wouldn't it be nice if infants and children wanted to sleep exactly where we wanted to put them on a given day? No joke here–it would be wonderful, but unfortunately it's not how most babies sleep. We've heard of mothers complaining about having to be outside walking for a nap to happen while living in cities with blizzards and 30 below weather, or needing to be walking constantly (inside or out), meaning naps are not only not a time of respite for mom, but can be downright unpleasant.

Interestingly, the most common situations involve touch, sound, or movement—three things that are abundant for the infant while in the womb. Recall that human babies are born at least 9 months early compared to other animals because of head size (if they got any bigger they could not get through the birth canal; see Trevathan, 2011), so for at least 9 months their bodies expect an "external womb."

So is it much of a surprise that outside the womb they expect the same things to lull them to sleep? With respect to **touch,** we know that oxytocin plays a huge role in feelings of contentment, security, and love, all of which affect the quality of our sleep (Uvnäs-Moberg, 2003). So it is not difficult to imagine that infants who are physically close to their caregivers, experiencing a release of oxytocin, are much more likely to fall asleep and remain asleep.

21

A second factor is **sound**–most notably the caregiver's heartbeat, a sound that is highly familiar to infants from their time in the womb. When it is the mother holding the infant, her heartbeat, voice, and breathing can all offer a form of white noise, which helps an infant feel safe and remain asleep, though the same effects can happen when another caregiver holds the infant as well.

When this is not possible, the use of a white noise machine to block out some of the more abrasive sounds of our environment while still providing background noise can help with infant sleep. These white noise machines have been successful in inducing infant sleep (Spencer, Moran, Lee, & Talbert, 1990), and at assisting some parents achieve better sleep (Lee & Gay, 2011).

The third factor, **movement**, was also abundant in the womb, with baby in a soft, liquid pouch being swayed regularly. Remember how your baby was always awake in utero when you were resting? It's because he or she was sleeping while you moved. Modern parents in Western cultures often focus on the car ride to get their infants to sleep. The lull of the car coupled with the snugness of the car seat can send many infants into a drowsy state, allowing them to nap contently while parents drive aimlessly around.

However, the same movement-induced sleep can be gained from the use of a stroller, providing mom or dad with the ability to run errands, or go for a walk or run. Possibly best of all, babywearing promotes movement, touch, and sound, all while allowing the caregiver to run errands, and generally go about one's life. Babywearing may provide the best form of an "external womb" for developing the baby's brain and body in optimal ways (Narvaez et al., 2013).

The take-home point, though, is *that it is normal for infants to prefer to sleep in contact with others rather than away from what many people would consider the "ideal" sleep space.* Even though adults may prefer it, a bed in a quiet room is not necessarily ideal for infant naps.

A Final Summary

We hope we have made it clear that often what parents perceive to be problematic infant sleep patterns that require "fixing" are actually quite normal and developmentally appropriate. We are cognizant of the fact that many families still find infant and toddler sleep to be a problem, which is why we are also focusing on writing about how to gently help with infant and toddler sleep.

What we hope parents take home is (a) a better understanding of the broad array of behaviors that constitute "normal" when it comes to our children's sleep, and (b) that if the behavior is not posing a problem for the family, you can rest assured the child is not suffering from these very normal sleep behaviors. Instead of following a particular expert's advice, understand what is needed to keep babies safe when they sleep and build the sleep environment around these safe behaviors. Then do what works best for your child.

Let your child be your guide.

References

Anders, T.F., Halpern, L.F., & Hua, J. (1992). Sleeping through the night: A developmental perspective. *Pediatrics, 90,* 554-560.

Ball, H. L. (2003). Breastfeeding, bed-sharing, and infant sleep. *Birth, 30,* 181-188.

Ball, H. L. (2009). Bed-sharing and co-sleeping: Research overview. *NCT New Digest, 48,* 22-27.

Barajas, R.G., Martin, A., Brooks-Gunn, J., & Hale, L. (2011). Mother-child bed-sharing in toddlerhood and cognitive and behavioral outcomes. *Pediatrics, 128,* e339-e347.

Butte, N. F., Jensen, C. L., Moon, J. K., Glaze, D. G., & Frost Jr., J. D. (1992). Sleep organization and energy expenditure of breast-fed and formula-fed infants. *Pediatric Research, 32,* 514-519.

Cassels, T.G. (2013). ADHD, sleep problems, and bed sharing: Future considerations. *The American Journal of Family Therapy, 41,* 13-25.

Delgado, P.L. (2006). Monoamine depletion studies: Implications for antidepressant discontinuation syndrome. *Journal of Clinical Psychiatry, 67*(4), 22-26.

Doan, T., Gardiner, A., Gay, C. L., & Lee, K. A. (2007). Breast-feeding increases sleep duration of new parents. *Journal of Perinatal & Neonatal Nursing, 21,* 200-206.

Elias, M. F., Nicolson, N. A., Bora, C., & Johnston, J. (1986). Sleep/wake patterns of breast-fed infants in the first 2 years of life. *Pediatrics, 77,* 322-329.

Goldman, A. S. (1993). The immune system of human milk: Antimicrobial anti-inflammatory and immunomodulating properties. *Pediatric Infectious Disease Journal, 12*(8), 664-671.

Goodlin-Jones, B. L., Burnham, M. M., Gaylor, E. E., & Anders, T. F. (2001). Night waking, sleep-wake organization, and self-soothing in the first year of life. *Journal of Developmental and Behavioral Pediatrics, 22*(4), 226.

Hibberd, C.M., Brooke, O.G., Carter, N.D., Haug, M., & Harzer, G. (1981). Variation in the composition of breast milk during the first five weeks of lactation: implications for the feeding of preterm infants. *Archives of Diseases of Childhood, 57,* 658-662.

Kendall-Tackett, K. A., Cong, Z., & Hale, T. W. (2011). The effect of feeding method on sleep duration, maternal well-being, and postpartum depression. *Clinical Lactation, 2*(2), 22-26.

Lee, K.A. & Gay, C.L. (2011). Can modifications to the bedroom environment improve the sleep of new parents? Two randomized control trials. *Research in Nursing and Health, 34,* 7-19.

Lien, E.L. (2003). Infant formulas with increased concentrations of α-lactalbumin. *American Journal of Clinical Nutrition, 77*(6), 1555S-1558S.

Loutzenhiser, L., Ahlquist, A., & Hoffman, J. (2011). Infant and maternal factors associated with maternal perceptions of infant sleep problems. *Journal of Reproductive and Infant Psychology, 29*(5), 460-471.

Matricciani, L. A., Olds, T. S., Blunden, S., Rigney, G., & Williams, M. T. (2012). Never enough sleep: A brief history of sleep recommendations for children. *Pediatrics, 129*, 548-556.

Meltzer, L.J., & Mindell, J.A. (2006). Sleep and sleep disorders in children and adolescents. *Psychiatric Clinics of North America, 29*, 1059-1076.

Messmer, R., Miller, L.D., & Yu, C.M. (2012). The relationship between parent-infant bed sharing and marital satisfaction for mothers of infants. *Family Relations, 61*, 798-810.

Middlemiss, W. (2004). Infant sleep: A review of normative and problematic sleep and interventions. *Early Child Development and Care, 174*, 99-122.

Mindell, J. A., Sadeh, A., Wiegand, B., How, T. H., & Goh, D. Y. T. (2010). Cross-cultural differences in infant and toddler sleep. *Sleep Medicine, 11*, 274-280.

Mindell, J. A., Telofski, L. S., Weigand, B., & Kurtz, E. S. (2009). A nightly bedtime routine: Impact on sleep in young children and maternal mood. *Sleep, 32*, 599-606.

Mosko, S., Richard, C., & McKenna, J. (1997). Infant arousals during mother-infant bed sharing: Implications for infant sleep and sudden infant death syndrome. *Pediatrics, 100*, 841-849.

Mosko, S., Richard, C., McKenna, J., & Drummond, S. (1996). Infant sleep architecture during bedsharing and possible implications for SIDS. *Sleep, 19*, 677-684.

Narvaez, D., Panksepp, J., Schore, A., & Gleason, T. (Eds.) (2013). *Evolution, early experience and human development: From research to practice and policy.* New York: Oxford University Press.

Nelson, E.A.S., & Taylor, B.J. (2001). International child care practices study: infant sleeping environment. *Early Human Development, 62*, 43-55.

Richman, N. (1981a). A community survey of characteristics of one to two-year-olds with sleep disruptions. *Journal of the American Academy of Child Psychiatry, 20*, 281-291.

Richman, N. (1981b). Sleep problems in young children. *Archives of Disease in Childhood, 56*, 491-493.

Scher, A. (1991). A longitudinal study of night waking in the first year. *Child: Care, Health and Development, 17*, 295-302.

Scher, A. (2001). Attachment and sleep: A study of night-waking in 12-month-old infants. *Developmental Psychobiology, 38*, 274-285.

Scher, A., Epstein, R., & Tirosh, E. (2004). Stability and changes in sleep regulation: A longitudinal study from 3 months to 3 years. *International Journal of Behavioral Development, 28*, 268-274.

Somer, E. (2009). *Eat your way to happiness.* New York: Harlequin.

Spencer, J.A., Moran, D.J., Lee, A., & Talbert, D. (1990). White noise and sleep induction. *Archives of Diseases in Childhood, 65*, 135-137.

Trevathan, W.R. (2011). *Human birth: An evolutionary perspective.* New York: Aldine de Gruyter.

Uvnäs-Moberg, K. (2003). *The oxytocin factor: Tapping the hormone of calm, love and healing.* Cambridge, MA: Da Capo Press.

Weinraub, M., Bender, R. H., Friedman, S. L., Susman, E. J., Knoke, B., Bradley, R., Houts, R., & Williams, J. (2012). Patterns of developmental change in infants' nighttime sleep awakenings from 6 through 36 months of age. *Developmental Psychology, 48*, 1511-1528.

Welles-Nystrom, B. (2005). Co-sleeping as a window into Swedish culture: considerations of gender and health care. *Scandinavian Journal of Caring Science, 19,* 354-360.

2

Simple Ways to Calm a Crying Baby And Have a More Peaceful Night's Sleep

Darcia Narvaez, Wendy Middlemiss,

John Hoffman, Helen Stevens, James McKenna,

Kathleen Kendall-Tackett, Tracy Cassels,

Sarah Ockwell-Smith

"My baby is only happy in my arms. The minute I put her down she cries."

"She wakes every hour throughout the night, every night. I'm exhausted."

Most Infants Wake at Night and Expect Comfort from their Parents

The number of times infants wake and need help to return to sleep decreases as they grow, but still remains fairly common. Recent research by Weinraub and her colleagues confirms how *normal it is for babies to wake at night*, with 66% of 6-month-olds still waking at least once or twice a week, and the remaining babies waking even more often. Some babies will cry when waking at 12 months of age—even babies who have settled back to sleep on other nights.

Helping an infant return to sleep easily, then, is an essential gift to give our infants, and an important goal for parents who need to rest. The science of nighttime care provides a good foundation for parents trying to calm their babies. It clarifies what is important to know about calming babies, and why certain types of calming are most likely to be helpful.

What Is Important to Know about Calming

A parent's presence helps to calm babies who awaken in an upset state

Babies (especially in the first few months) are not yet capable of regulating their emotional states. This is one of the reasons why crying tends to increase in the first 2 to 3 months of life, and then decrease steadily after that. Infants cry or fuss for many reasons, including hunger, pain, or other discomforts or, at times, simply a desire for physical contact.

For example, infant crying/fussing behavior generally decreases by as much as 43% at 6 weeks of age (Hunziker & Barr, 1988).

Fussing and crying are the most important means by which an infant communicates needs and desires. The specific reason cannot always be determined, but for sure, displaying visible and audible signs of distress is an infant's most important defense and is overwhelmingly adaptive. When upset, babies depend on sensory input from caregivers—touch, soothing voice, smell, eye gaze, breastfeeding—in order to calm down. That's the way nature designed it to work.

Babies rely on their caregivers to calm them and to help deal with other reasons they are unhappy or uncomfortable, such as being in pain, hungry, or in some sort of physical or emotional state that we can't determine. Being present and attending to infants when they wake and cry can help infants return to sleep more quickly (Mao, Burnham, Goodlin-Jones, Gaylor, & Anders, 2004).

Calming infants helps infants learn to calm themselves

By helping infants calm down by attending to their distress, caregivers help infants develop the tools—both physiologically and emotionally—to calm themselves. This is what parents help children with generally (Davidov & Grusec, 2006; Stifter & Spinrad,

2002). Parents are often hesitant to be present when babies cry, fearing that attending to crying babies will lead babies to be unable to deal with distress on their own. But this approach only leads to a fussy baby and a clingy child.

Leaving babies to cry increases babies' stress levels and often keeps them awake longer. It does not guide them emotionally or physically toward the goal of regulating their own distress and response. Instead, to develop "good" or "healthy" sleep habits, gentle parental guidance is needed to resettle. Over time this leads to a strong, self-settling child who can calm him or herself when challenges arise.

Bottom Line

Crying upon waking is a perfectly normal behavior. Helping crying infants feel comforted and calm supports their developing abilities to calm themselves over time.

Understand why some babies fuss more at night than other babies

Fussing upon awakening is a perfectly normal behavior. When babies are distressed they are indicating a need for attention, often to help them recover a feeling of security. It is, however, important to understand that babies differ in what makes them feel secure.

Because some infants don't cry very much or very forcefully, some people develop the expectation that all babies can/should be like that. But babies vary greatly in terms of how often and how hard they cry. These differences are driven by many factors, including temperament, experience and physiological maturity. Thus, the need for external regulation (calming) continues in varying degrees for different babies.

Providing external regulation for babies who feel less secure, and thus more distressed, actually *helps* them, not hinders them. It helps them build the neural pathways that eventually enable them to deal with stress and calm themselves (Cassidy, 1994; Stifter & Spinrad, 2002).

Understand when waking is a problem

Waking is a normal part of infant sleep, and varies based on several infant factors: (a) feeding method (breast or bottle), (b) age, (c) shifts in developmental levels, and (d) individual level of maturity. In light of these factors, every family must determine whether an infants' waking is a problem for the family. Waking isn't a problem just because it happens. To suggest waking defines "problematic sleep" does not accurately reflect current science.

We know that it is normal for infants to wake several times in the night, especially if breastfeeding. And given that human babies are neurologically immature at birth, awakenings are the infants' major line of defense against dangerous, prolonged breathing pauses and permits oxygenation. Moreover, transient and more prolonged awakenings can help respond to cardiopulmonary challenges while asleep and restore a more natural heart rhythmicity (Mosko et al., 1997a).

Recall that the early research on sudden infant death syndrome (SIDS) revealed that infants who woke frequently in the night were less likely to die of SIDS than those who awakened significantly less often (see review in McKenna 1995 and Mosko et al., 1997a and b).

Even then it may be more helpful to frame the night waking as a family problem rather than as a child's "sleep problem." If a parent is OK with a baby waking two or more times a night at 12 months then there is no problem!

After babies are beyond the age of chief risk for SIDS, and their waking and sleeping is settling into more of a consistent pattern, research shows that many continue to wake in the night (Weinraub et al., 2012).

Calming Ways to Calm Babies

The first 3 months of life is known to many as "The Fourth Trimester" and requires similar care to the womb. Some babies make the womb-to-world transition easily, others less so. Many of the ways parents naturally try to calm babies actually re-create many of the comforting, familiar experiences infants had during their time in utero. For all babies, these calming techniques can be very comforting.

Parents can help recreate these calming environments across any sleep routine and sleep pattern. It's important to remember what is calming and why.

Recreate movement

The womb is a constantly moving space and babies tend to respond by calming to movements, such as dancing, swaying from side to side, going for an exaggerated quick walk, or bumpy car ride.

Rely on touch; Provide skin-to-skin contact

Being in contact with warm, naturally (un)scented, skin is proved to be calming for infants/babies, it helps to stabilize their body temperature, heart rate, and stress hormones, and stimulates the release of oxytocin—the love and bonding hormone–in parent and baby both.

Recreate familiar sounds

The babies' time in the womb was marked by many rhythmic sounds. Sounds similar to those babies heard in the womb can be very calming. White noise offers constant surrounding sounds while also slowing brain wave frequencies.

Help the infant learn to deal with sensations of hunger

Hunger is a new sensation for infants—and infants may find it hard to calm when they feel hungry. Feeding babies when they wake at night can help babies transition back to sleep, especially when lighting and interaction are kept at low levels of stimulation.

Babies also find sucking to be the ultimate relaxation and comfort tool, one of their few forms of self-initiated self-regulation. Sucking helps a baby's skull bones to return to their normal position after birth as well as providing them with comfort and security. Some infants/babies respond to sucking on a dummy/pacifier as soothing (but avoid this in the early weeks of breastfeeding as it can pose problems establishing breastfeeding). Non-nutritive suckling on the breast is also calming.

Parents can help recreate these calming environments across any sleep routine and sleep pattern. It's important to remember what is calming and why.

Sleep Routines that Can Help Calm Babies

Keep babies close

Keeping babies close helps in shared breathing, touch, warmth, and awareness of any difficulties. Babies are generally much calmer and sleep more easily if they are sleeping with their caregivers, or in very close proximity.

Babies can benefit from the shared breathing (and general sensory exchanges) with the caregiver including skin-to-skin contact, and this can be achieved to varying degrees depending on the overall safety conditions, including keeping the infant on a separate surface next to your bed, a behavior called separate-surface *co-sleeping*.

Many breastfeeding mothers find that intermittent *bedsharing* helps them continue breastfeeding, especially if they work during the day. Bedsharing (while the American Academy of Pediatrics currently recommends against it) not only increases sleep time both for mothers and babies, but has the effect of increasing the chances that mothers will breastfeed for a greater number of months than if they place their infant elsewhere for sleep.

Close proximity usually means night feeds are much easier, there are more of them, and they are far less disruptive for parents and infants, and thus can be more settling. That said, just as with any sleep arrangement, bedsharing does carry risks (as does sleeping away from the baby), and there are very clear circumstances that we know that make bedsharing not advisable.

When bedsharing should be avoided

Bedsharing should be avoided if mothers smoked during pregnancy, because infant arousal patterns may not be as efficient as they should be for maximum safety in a bedsharing environment. The same holds true for small premature infants. They are safest sleeping alongside the bed in a different sleep structure rather than in the bed. And, finally, it is highly risky to fall asleep with an infant on a couch, sofa, or armchair, as many infants have suffocated by being trapped between the adult and some part of the furniture. In all these cases, co-sleeping (different surface, same room) is more advisable than bedsharing. In any sleep location, infants must be placed on their backs to sleep.

It is important for the caregivers to refrain from bedsharing if they are not breastfeeding, and obviously if any adult is under the influence of alcohol, drugs, or anything that may impair their natural arousal patterns. Surely, babies should sleep alongside the bed on a different surface: (a) if adult bedsharers are excessively sleepy, (b) if smaller children are likely to find their way into the parents' bed, or (c) if there is another adult present in bed who refuses to take any responsibility for the infant.

Finally, wherever infants sleep they should always be placed on their backs. Moreover, if sleeping with or away from caregivers, infants should be positioned away from soft bedding, pillows, or toys and be situated so that breathing is never obstructed, with their heads never covered.

Breastfeed

In addition to all its other associated benefits to infant health and cognitive development, breastfeeding is an excellent way to calm a baby. It provides skin-to-skin contact and warmth. Breastfeeding can be of benefit to the caregiver as well, making wakings easier to manage and helping to reduce postpartum depression (Dennis & McQueen, 2009; Fergerson, Jamieson, & Lindsay, 2002; Kendall-Tackett, 2007).

In one recent study, mothers who exclusively breastfed actually got more sleep and were less tired during the day than mothers who either exclusively formula fed or both breast- and formula-fed (Kendall-Tackett, Cong, & Hale, 2011).

Listen to the baby and trust your caring instincts

Babies are master communicators, just as adults typically are masters at figuring out how best to respond. Adults don't learn to rock a baby or to talk softly— these come naturally. So to calm babies, it is helpful to follow the baby's lead and follow one's heart. Parents need to learn to follow their hearts and keep babies safe and healthy. If holding the baby seems to cause distress, then parents can stay with them, but place them in a position that seems more helpful. If the parent is still, perhaps walk; if the parent is already moving, perhaps rock. Parents should trust their instincts in how to be present with the baby.

What If the Routine Is Still Stressful?

A time may come when a parent starts thinking, "I've been doing nighttime comforting for quite awhile now. Is there anything I can do to move towards getting some uninterrupted nights?"

The answer is yes. Partly, it comes with time—varying times for different babies as Weinraub's recent study showed. And there are some things parents can do to gently move in that direction with the baby. We will share some ways to help babies need less attention at night, if that is something that is essential for a family's well-being. These approaches will build on the essential steps for calming discussed here:

Listen to the baby's signals.

Provide nurturance and support.

Help babies help themselves calm.

Remember, there is only one expert in caring for your baby—you. Sometimes you will find a way to calm your baby easily. Sometimes it may seem like what worked before doesn't work now. Being patient with your baby and yourself will help you both learn and grow.

References

Cassidy, J. (1994). Emotion regulation: Influences of attachment relationships. *Monographs of the Society for Research in Child Development, 59,* 228-283.

Davidov, M., & Grusec, J.E. (2006). Untangling the links of parental responsiveness to distress and warmth to child outcomes. *Child Development, 77,* 44-58.

Dennis, C.-L., & McQueen, K. (2009). The relationship between infant-feeding outcomes and postpartum depression: A qualitative systematic review. *Pediatrics, 123,* e736-e751.

Fergerson, S.S., Jamieson, D.J., & Lindsay, M. (2002). Diagnosing postpartum depression: Can we do better? *American Journal of Obstetrics and Gynecology,* 186, 899-902.

Hunziker, U.A., & Barr, R.G. (1986). Increased carrying reduces infant crying: A randomized controlled trial. *Pediatrics, 77,* 641-648. ftp://urstm.com/CharestJ/Articles. pdf/Hunziker%20U%201986.pdf

Kendall-Tackett, K. A. (2007). A new paradigm for depression in new mothers: The central role of inflammation and how breastfeeding and anti-inflammatory treatments protect maternal mental health. *International Breastfeeding Journal,* 2:6 http://www.internationalbreastfeeding-journal.com/content/2/1/6

Kendall-Tackett, K.A., Cong, Z., & Hale, T.W. (2011). The effect of feeding method on sleep duration, maternal well-being, and postpartum depression. *Clinical Lactation, 2*(2), 22-26.

Mao, A., Burnham, M.M., Goodlin-Jones, B.L., Gaylor, E.E., & Anders T.F. (2004). A comparison of the sleep-wake patterns of cosleeping and solitary-sleeping infants. *Child Psychiatry and Human Development, 35,* 95-105.

McKenna, J.J. (1995). The potential benefits of infant-parent co-sleeping in relation to SIDS prevention. In T. O. Rognum (Ed.), *Sudden Infant Death Syndrome: New trends in the nineties* (pp. 257-265). Oslo, Norway: Scandinavian Press.

McKenna, J.J., & Mosko, S. (1990). Evolution and the sudden infant death syndrome (SIDS) Part II: Why human infants? *Human Nature, 1* (2), 145-177.

McKenna, J.J., & Mosko, S. (1990). Evolution and the sudden infant death syndrome (SIDS), Part III: Parent-infant co-sleeping and infant arousal, *Human Nature, 1*(2), 145-177.

McKenna, J.J., & Mosko, S. (2001). Mother-infant cosleeping: Toward a new scientific beginning. In R. Byard & H. Krous, (Eds.), *Sudden Infant Death Syndrome: Puzzles, problems and possibilities*. London: Arnold Publishers.

Mosko, S., Richard, C., & McKenna, J. (1997). Infant arousals during mother-infant bed sharing: Implications for infant Sleep and SIDS research. *Pediatrics, 100*(2), 841-849.

Mosko, S., Richard, C., & McKenna, J. (1997). Maternal sleep and arousals during bedsharing with infants. *Sleep, 201*(2), 142-150.

Stifter, C.A., & Spinrad, T.L. (2002). The effect of excessive crying on the development of emotion regulation. *Infancy, 3*, 133-152.

Weinraub, M., Bender, R.H., Friedman, S.L., Susman, E.J., Knoke, B., Bradley, R., Houts, R., Williams, J. (2012). Patterns of developmental change in infants' nighttime sleep awakenings from 6 through 36 months of age. *Developmental Psychology, 48*, 1501-1528.

3

Bringing the Parent Back into Decisions about Nighttime Care

Wendy Middlemiss

New parents often have many questions and concerns about how to help their children grow strong and healthy. Unfortunately, when it comes to nighttime care, health care providers often tell parents what to do rather than discussing options. Health care providers might give parents specific advice about how to handle nighttime wakings, for example, without inquiring about parents' beliefs and preferences. When health care providers simply tell parents what to do, parents may choose to ignore the advice if it is not consistent with their beliefs and preferences. When parents and health care providers do not communicate, parents do not get the information they need to cope with some of the more challenging aspects of infancy, including nighttime waking.

This chapter presents information on how to bring parents back into decisions about nighttime care by discussing issues more broadly, addressing parents' concerns regarding responsiveness, and focusing on the essentials of infant safety and health. When professionals can have open discussions with parents, parents gain the tools they need to make decisions that best fit their families' needs.

What Is the Allure of Reducing Nightwaking?

Health care providers often make specific recommendations about nighttime care that focus on reducing nightwakings, creating solitary sleep settings for infants, and limiting parents' contact with infants during their transitions to sleep. These recommendations for nighttime infant care reflect many common components of "best practice" recommendations (Morgenthaler et al., 2006) and American Academy of Pediatrics policy recommendations (American Academy of Pediatrics, 2000; 2011).

However, recommendations can sometimes limit conversation about developmentally appropriate sleep routines, infant safety, and flexibility in parent choices.

Of importance then, in supporting parents in their early care decisions, is to find a balance between the essential aspects of best-practice and policy recommendations, and parents' role in the decision making regarding care. With this, professionals can help parents create sleep routines that are safe, incorporate best-practice approaches, and fit the family's childrearing preferences.

Finding this balance can be very important when discussing issues, such as nighttime wakings and infants' ability to settle to sleep, without parents' assistance or presence. In this chapter, support for different sleep approaches is examined—with an eye toward facilitating discussions between parents and professionals.

Benefit or Risk?

Helping infants learn to sleep through the night without parents' help or attention is a compelling sleep goal. Controlled crying is one way that parents can achieve this end. Some healthcare providers like sleep-training approaches because they can be both simple to discuss, and successful, can result in fewer nightwakings requiring parent attention, and have outcomes that are easy to quantify.

Unfortunately, this successful approach does not take into account breastfeeding, parental responsiveness, normal fluctuations in infant sleep patterns at different ages, infant emotional regulation, maturity of infant autonomic functioning, infant settling and safety, or the parents' cultural preferences.

With this approach, infants can be "trained" to settle to sleep, and wake and resettle, without parental assistance through behavioral sleep interventions. Parents can be encouraged to focus on the goal of sleep consolidation. But is this an appropriate goal?

Certainly nightwakings, particularly in the context of helping infants settle to sleep, can be challenging for new parents. When infants wake, parents do too. This can influence parents' quality of sleep and their parenting efforts (McDaniel & Teti, 2013). Reducing nightwakings, then, benefits parents by increasing the duration of both their sleep and their infants' sleep. Advocates of sleep training believe that the benefits of their approach clearly outweigh any potential costs (Price et al., 2012).

As noted in the previous section, however, the costs are far from negligible (see Miller & Commons and Narvaez, this volume). Infants can learn to settle themselves to sleep without parental assistance using behavioral-sleep interventions. However, even though infants stop crying for parents' attention, research has shown that infants continue to experience high levels of physiological distress (Middlemiss et al., 2012).

What this means is that infants appear to be able to settle to sleep without distress—which is very relieving for parents if their infants had been crying at nighttime. But infants are still experiencing distress even though they are no longer signaling that distress through crying. Considering that crying is an essential way for infants to communicate, the fact that they are no longer doing so is concerning.

This disconnect between infants' physiological experience of stress and their behavioral expression of this distress through crying is only one concern with behavioral approaches to nighttime care. There are other consequences when mothers are told to not respond to their babies' cries in order to eliminate nightwaking.

Non-responsive parenting may encourage mothers to establish routines that interfere with breastfeeding, and that do not support infants' biological and physiological development. Taken together as a whole, the cry-it-out approach gives mothers an inflexible set of baby-care rules that do not accommodate the normal fluctuations in breastfeeding, nightwakings, and infant growth.

Parents Become Less Comfortable Providing Infant Care

Thus, it is important to create discussions with parents that neither begin nor end with considerations of nightwakings. Childrearing is complicated, and there are many factors that contribute to its complexity. Mothers differ in their childcare preferences and the ease with which they transition to the role of caregiver.

In their recent study, Countermine and Teti (2010) examined a number of parenting factors, such as nighttime infant care, nightwakings, depression, and spousal agreement regarding infant care. They concluded that:

> The "best" sleep arrangements for infants may prove to be those that both parents are most comfortable with and that promote family harmony (p. 661).

Thus, rather than focusing on nightwakings—which is only one aspect of parenting—health care providers should help mothers find approaches that meet babies' needs and increase family well-being. Professionals can help parents make informed, comfortable choices about caring for their infants.

Is Comfort with Care That Important?

Recent research on parental adaptation, defined as parental comfort with their abilities as parents, suggests that parents are more effective when they are confident about their parenting skills (Countermine & Teti, 2010). Researchers have found that parents' comfort with providing care is important in many different contexts. In looking specifically at infant nighttime care and adaptation, research indicates that when parents report high levels of stress, they have lower levels of parental self-efficacy (Jones & Prinz, 2005).

When the parents are responsive to infants' needs, parental adaptation predicts higher levels of functioning and adjustment in children over time (Countermine & Teti, 2010). In sum, parents who are well adapted, and have lower levels of parental stress, are more responsive during nighttime care, and report better quality of sleep (Ramos & Youngclarke, 2006). And when mothers are adapted, their babies sleep better too (Countermine & Teti, 2010).

Working with Parents to Develop a Strategy for Nighttime Care

Professionals can help parents construct a system of care that meets their infants' needs, and is appropriate for their caregiving preferences. Parents feel respected when professionals listen to their concerns. When the practices health care providers recommend are consistent with parents' values and beliefs, parents are more likely to incorporate these practices into their parenting (Nobile & Drotar, 2003).

Rather than simply focus on reducing nightwakings, you can work with parents to come up with strategies that address infants', mothers', and families' needs. You can incorporate their values into the nighttime-care plan, while encouraging parents to know their infants and trust their instincts for care. You can also help them be comfortable with different approaches to care and help them understand that their babies need them at night, and that parents also benefit when they are available to meet their infants' needs.

Below are some strategies for parents to help them cope with nighttime care and adapt to parenthood.

Know Your Infant, Trust Your Instincts

One of the first steps is helping parents understand the nature of nighttime care and infants' developing and fluctuating sleep patterns. Sharing this information with parents helps focus on identifying realistic expectations and helping parents understand what is essential to their infants, their caregiving, and their childrearing goals.

With this refocusing of discussions about infant sleep, parents can ask questions about nighttime care choices and related benefits or risks. For example, do parents want to sleep in the same bed and breastfeed their infant? If they do, then conversations can address the benefits of breastfeeding and infant safe-sleep environments, as well as likely sleep patterns.

Do parents want infants to sleep through the night? If so, discussion can include how to help parents address this goal without compromising breastfeeding or infants' natural need for responsiveness and proximity. With this focus, responsiveness and breastfeeding are not considered within the framework of infant nightwakings.

Nighttime wakings and crying become a natural and expected part of the sleep routine—one to be discussed, but not to be the central focus. When parents are comfortable with their care choices, and feel efficacious and well adapted to their role as parents, everyone in the family benefits (Middlemiss, 2010).

One benefit is lower likelihood of physiological distress at nighttime (Middlemiss, 2010). Infants receive care that builds their regulatory, social, and physiological systems and reflects their specific developmental needs.

Mothers can feel confident that they are meeting their infants' needs, while still tending to their own mental health (Thome & Skulladottirr, 2005), and cooperating with their partners in parenting decisions (McDaniels & Teti, 2013).

Comfort with Adapting Care to Your Infants' Changing Patterns

By refocusing conversations on a diversity of acceptable nighttime-care practices (i.e., not only practices that may reduce nightwakings), parents can become comfortable with adapting their care to their infants' needs. When mothers accept that there are different care choices, they are more likely to be adapted to their care choice.

This was demonstrated in a recent study of mothers. Mothers who chose to co-sleep still had higher stress levels when initiating the nighttime care than mothers whose babies slept alone. These findings were due, in part, to higher levels of stress associated with feelings of being criticized for their nighttime-care choices (Middlemiss et al., 2009).

The co-sleeping mothers were asked why they were satisfied with their decision to co-sleep, yet still reported high levels of stress. These mothers indicated that they were uncomfortable because they knew that co-sleeping was generally not accepted. Their personal comfort with the routine was compromised by the sense that they were not taking care of their infant the way that they "should," i.e., in a manner that limited parental presence and focused on nightwakings.

The mothers discussed, at length, their preferences for shared-sleep routines and the benefits they believed their infants derived from this type of care. Yet because they had heard that solitary sleep was the "best practice," they were uncomfortable with their care choice (Middlemiss et al., 2009).

Panchula (2012) discussed the importance of helping mothers be comfortable with their care routines. She noted that families' cultural framework is an important component of the type of care that the family will receive. In supporting families, it is essential to help them find solutions to problems that fit within the mothers' cultural preferences and their current situation. She emphasized that listening to parents is an important first step to any intervention.

With this approach, parents feel comfortable expressing their preferences, and professionals can provide guidance in a manner that resonates with parents' childrearing goals.

Helping parents feel comfortable with their childrearing choices is essential to successfully providing support and usable information (Ball et al., 2013; Cowan, 2012; Moon et al., 2008)—information that supports both continued breastfeeding and infant safety. Professionals can assure parents that nightwaking is often a normal sleep pattern for infants and toddlers.

Infants' sleep varies by how they are fed; whether parents are present while they sleep; and individual variables, such as temperament, prematurity, or well-being. All of these variables influence the nature and quality of infant sleep.

In their work, Thome and colleagues (2005) found that sharing information about normal infant sleep can have a positive impact on mothers' mental health.

Flexibility in Your Choices of Care

Mothers who wanted their infants to settle to sleep alone were less stressed when they were flexible with their care routines. In a study of infant sleep location, mothers who had firm beliefs about where babies should sleep were more stressed when they placed their infants in bed than mothers who were more flexible about sleep arrangements. Interestingly, this finding was true for both mothers who preferred that their infants sleep alone and mothers who believed they should be present while their infants slept (Yaure et al., 2011).

Mothers in both groups with flexible care routines (i.e., remaining with infants until they had fallen asleep and then placing them down) had lower levels of stress. This was even true for mothers who preferred that their infants have solitary, self-settling routines. This flexibility in routine can be helpful for parents as infants' patterns of sleep fluctuate with developmental changes, illnesses, and other factors.

With this flexibility, professionals are better positioned to help parents incorporate continued breastfeeding into their nighttime care choices—a choice that is ultimately of great benefit for both infant and mother.

Maternal flexibility has long-term effects. One of our studies explored the association between mothers' comfort with the sleep routine their 5-year-olds had as infants, and their ratings of their children's social competencies. Mothers' comfort with their care practices was related to their children's social competency at age 5 years. Parental presence vs. self-settling was not (Middlemiss et al., 2002).

Sorting Out the Quandary of Remaining Present with Infants and Nightwakings

When professionals focus on how to best support breastfeeding and mother/infant sleep, they no longer need to focus solely on infant sleep location. This can help support parents in making choices that best fit their family and personal needs, as well as their infants' needs. For example, many parents prefer to be present during infants' nighttime routines, particularly as they transition to sleep (St. James-Roberts, 2007). This preference has been reported even for mothers focused on encouraging infant self-settling (Morgenthaler et al., 2006).

However, sometimes parents feel that they must choose between continued breastfeeding—often inclusive of nightwakings—or helping their infants learn self-settling routines. Self-soothing infants settle without parental assistance and sleep in locations portrayed to be the most safe.

If health care providers do not discuss benefits and risks of various sleep locations, parents may feel that the only two options are bedsharing or letting their babies cry in another room. To facilitate mothers' adaptation to care and comfort with their care choices, health care providers must share information regarding different approaches to nighttime care and their benefits for families and infants. In the next section are some aspects of care that support choices across care routines.

Assurances of Infant Safety across Routines

Many parents prefer to remain with their infants during their transition to sleep, and many prefer to share sleep or bedshare. However, messages regarding the potential risk for infants in shared settings can lead parents to make choices that they do not feel comfortable with.

In making their decisions about nighttime care, parents may inadvertently introduce unnecessary risk in the nighttime routines. For example, proximity at night, although associated with more parental awareness of nightwakings, has been linked to an increase in response to infant distress, reducing infant stress reactivity, thus reducing this risk factor for future psychopathology (Tollenar et al., 2012).

Providing parents with information about safe infant sleep is critical. But such information needs to move beyond scare tactics and be more nuanced about what makes infant sleep healthy. It is important to assure parents that breastfeeding has been shown to reduce the risk of SIDS, particularly when bedsharing (AAP, 2011; McKenna, 2007).

Breastfeeding while bedsharing places infants in a safe position from which they are least likely to roll over to an unsafe position. A study examining mother-and-infant sleep environments found mothers engaged in different methods of protecting infants across different sleep settings (Volpe, Ball, & McKenna, 2013). Thus, discussions of safe infant sleep need to address different sleep practices.

When information about infant safety is not provided within the context of preference for care, infants' risks increase. Information is not heard as applicable to parents based on their choices for care (Moon et al., 2012).

The essentials of infant sleep are not discussed and parents often are left to ignore both the essential components of care protective of infants and the components of care that do not fit within their family system. Because infant safety can be assured across a diversity of sleep settings, sharing information about parents' preferred care routine is essential.

Understanding the Value of Responsiveness and Presence

Part of the quandary regarding nighttime care comes from the general sense that being present during nighttime care harms infants and keeps them from developing healthy sleep routines. Parents are particularly concerned that being present for their infants will lead to more nightwakings and poorer infant sleep. It is important, then, to assure parents that responsiveness is essential and help parents incorporate responsiveness within their preferred sleep routines. This may be the first step to helping parents establish and maintain breastfeeding across nighttime care.

Perceiving cries as needing attention has been found to be an important factor in mothers' response (Middlemiss et al., 2009). Mothers least likely to perceive infants' cries as needing attention were less likely to attend to infants. This lack of response, however, was associated with infants experiencing higher levels of physiological stress during their transition to sleep in comparison to infants whose mothers perceived their cries as indicating distress.

The value of responsiveness moves beyond that of its developmentally appropriate nature in supporting infants' development. Parents who respond to their infants' cries have higher levels of adaptation to parenting during nighttime care (Teti et al., 2010), and greater parental efficacy in comparison to parents who did not respond to their babies and practiced sleep training and other parental-sleep routines (Countermine & Teti, 2010).

When parents ignored their babies' cries as a means of reducing nightwakings, it was problematic for parents and infants (France & Blampied, 2005; Morgenthaler et al., 2006). Not responding to infants' cries also led to higher levels of infant stress (Yaure et al., 2011). Telling parents about the benefits of responsive parenting can help them feel good about their parenting choices and/or help them be flexible in their nighttime parenting approaches.

Summary and Conclusions

What does this research on infant-sleep practices mean, then, for practice? Perhaps of greatest import is the message that mothers' comfort with and adaptation to the role of care provider is essential to helping families transition to parenting.

By talking to parents about nighttime care practices in general, rather than focusing only on night-wakings, lactation consultants become guides who both share information with parents and gather information from them. In helping mothers establish early-care routines, you can actually support mothers, rather than "supporting" them by focusing on infants sleeping through the night, scheduled feedings, and other means of controlling a routine or schedule.

These interventions, even when successful in the short term, may have high costs. You can support mothers by helping them understand the importance of knowing and having a relationship with their infants, and how to balance infant care with providing for their own needs. With a broader focus on normal infant sleep behavior, and realistic expectations for early care, parents can have a clearer understanding, and be more knowledgeable and accepting as they establish healthy and appropriate care routines.

Parents often anticipate that the "terrible twos"—whether terrible or not so bad—will be a time of toddlers proving that they are "able to do it by themselves." Adolescence can be a time of conflict between parents and teens. So it follows that infancy can be a time marked by nightwakings, and that responsiveness is important to meeting these care needs. Thus, in working with new parents, it is important to help them understand that there are many times infants will wake, and that there are many options for care.

What may be most helpful is to let parents know that early nighttime care can be a challenging time, when parents are tired and sometimes frustrated or flustered. Discuss with parents what to expect, and how they can meet their babies' needs. This can provide parents with the assurance that they can find "their" best way to parent.

The role of the professional is essential in providing parents with the tools to establish their routines, to meet the changes and challenges, and to be comfortable with how their care will provide a strong foundation for their child's developing emotional well-being, physical well-being, and brain.

References

American Academy of Pediatrics Task Force on Infant Sleep Position and Sudden Infant Death (2000). Changing concepts of sudden infant death syndrome: Implications for infant sleeping environment and sleep position. *Pediatrics, 105,* 650-656.

American Academy of Pediatrics, & Task Force on Sudden Infant Death Syndrome. (2011). Policy Statement: SIDS and other sleep-related deaths: Expansion of recommendations for a safe infant sleeping environment. *Pediatrics, 128*(5), 1030-1039.

Ball, H.L., & Volpe, L. (2013), Sudden Infant Death Syndrome (SIDS) risk reduction and infant sleep location—Moving the discussion forward. *Social Science & Medicine, 79,* 84-91.

Countermine, M.S., & Teti, D.M. (2010). Sleep arrangements and maternal adaptation in infancy. *Infant Mental Health Journal, 31*(6), 647–663. DOI: 10.1002/imhj.20276

Cowan, S. (2012). Creating change: How knowledge translates into action for protecting babies from Sudden Infant Death? *Current Pediatric Reviews, 6,* 86-94.

McDaniel, D.T., & Teti D. M. (2013). Coparenting quality during the first three months after birth: The role of infant sleep quality. *Journal of Family Psychology, 26,* 886-895.

McKenna, J. J., Mosko, S. S., & Richard, C. A. (1997), Bedsharing promotes breastfeeding. *Pediatrics, 100,* 214–219.

Meijer, A.M. (2011). Infant sleep consolidation: New perspectives. *Sleep Medicine Reviews, 15,* 209–210. doi:10.1016/j.smrv.2011.01.004

Middlemiss, W., Granger, D.A., Goldberg, W.A., & Nathans, L. (2012). Asynchrony of mother–infant hypothalamic–pituitary–adrenal axis activity following extinction of infant responses induced during the transition to sleep. *Early Human Development, 88,* 227-232. doi:10.1016/j. earlhumdev.2011.08.010

Middlemiss, W. (2010, August). *Working with families through a process orientation: Focusing on best practices through family strengths.* Invited paper presented at the International Scholar Series at Ewha Woman's University, Seoul, Korea.

Middlemiss, W. (2005). Prevention and intervention: Using resiliency-based multisetting approaches and a process-orientation. *Child and Adolescent Social Work Journal, 22,* 85-103.

Middlemiss, W. (2004a). Infant sleep: A review of normative and problematic sleep and interventions. *Early Child Development and Care, 174*(1), 99-122. doi:10.1080/0300443032000153516

Middlemiss, W. (2004b) Work in progress: Defining problematic infant sleep: Shifting the focus from deviance to difference. *Zero to Three, 24,* 46-51.

Moon, R. Y., Calabrese, T., & Aird, L. (2008). Reducing the risk of Sudden Infant Death Syndrome in child care and changing provider practices: Lessons learned from a demonstration project. *Pediatrics, 122,* 788-798.

Nobile, C., & Drotar, D. (2003). Research on the quality of parent-provider communication in pediatric care: Implications and recommendations. *Journal of Developmental & Behavioral Pediatrics, 24*(4), 279-290.

Panchula, J. (2012). Working with families of different cultures I. Lessons learned. *Clinical Lactation, 3*(1), 13-15.

Price, A.M.H, Wake, M., Ukoumunne, O.C., & Hiscock, H. (2012). Outcomes at six years of age for children with infant sleep problems: Longitudinal community-based study. *Sleep Medicine, 13,* 991-998. doi: 10.1016/j. sleep.2012.04.014

Sadeh, A., Tikotsky, L., & Scher, A. (2010). Parenting and infant sleep. *Sleep Medicine Review, 14,* 89-96

St. James-Roberts, I. (2007). Infant crying and sleeping: Helping parents to prevent and manage problems. *Sleep Medicine Clinics,* 2(3), 363-375, DOI: 10.1016/j.jsmc.2007.05.015.

Teti, D.M., & Crosby, B. (2012). Maternal depressive symptoms, dysfunctional cognitions, and infant night waking: The role of maternal nighttime behavior. *Child Development, 83,* 939–953. DOI: 10.1111/j.1467-8624.2012.01760.x

Teti, D.M., Kim, B.-R., Mayer, G., & Countermine, M. (2010). Maternal emotional availability at bedtime predicts infant sleep quality. *Journal of Family Psychology, 24*(3), 307-315. doi: 10.1037/a0019306

Thome, M., & Skulladottir, A. (2005). Evaluating a family-centered intervention of infant sleep problems. *Journal of Advanced Nursing, 50,* 5-11.

Volpe, L. E., Ball, H. L., & McKenna, J. J. (2013). Nighttime parenting strategies and sleep-related risks to infants. *Social Science & Medicine, 79,* 92-100.

Yaure, R., Middlemiss, W., & Huey, E. (2011, November). *Infant nighttime care: What should we consider?* Paper presented at the National Council on Family Relations Annual Conference, Orlando, FL.

4

We Go Together Like ...
Breastfeeding and
Cosleeping

Tracy Cassels

"100 years of rapidly changing infant-care fashions cannot alter several million years of evolutionarily derived infant physiology."

Helen Ball

Sleep and feeding have become two of the most discussed and disseminated topics in parenting today. How much sleep are you getting? Do you use formula or just the breast? When should a child sleep through the night? Do you pump? Does dad feed the little one at all? Do you room-share, bedshare, or put the little one alone in his room? What about sex?

There is an endless array of questions and judgments and "shoulds" associated with both infant sleep and feeding. But this hasn't always been the case. It used to be a simple matter of mother breastfeeding, and mother and infant sleeping together with no judgment and no questions about quality or quantity of sleep. For this reason, breastfeeding and co-sleeping are huge parts of evolutionary parenting; they facilitate the bond between mother and infant via skin-to-skin contact (Uvnas-Moberg, 2003), co-sleeping works to keep baby's temperature and breathing regulated (Ball, Blair, & Ward-Platt, 2004; McKenna & McDade, 2005), and it seems to provide parents and baby with better sleep (McKenna, Ball, & Gettler, 2007), while breastfeeding offers vital immune protection to infants necessary for survival (Duijts, Jaddoe, Hofman, & Moll, 2010).

Where Babies Sleep and How They Feed

For most mothers in contemporary Western societies, breastfeeding and infant sleeping arrangements are two distinct parenting practices with little or no relation to one another. To talk about one is not to talk about the other. Biologically, however, the two are inextricably intertwined.

For much of human history, Hunter-Gatherer societies dominated and in this domain, women were as central to the survival of the clan as men. There were no maternity leaves, but the work done by women was of the less-dangerous gatherer type, meaning they were able to do their work with children and infants in tow.

But with this came the necessity for women to sleep well, as a woman who is sleep-deprived does not serve anyone well in any capacity (it is truly strange that we have adopted the modern view that sleep deprivation is a "normal" state of affairs with a newborn).

As for the infant, without any alternatives, they required their mother's breast milk to survive, much less thrive. And thus we reach the point at which breastfeeding and cosleeping collide—in order to breastfeed continuously without immense sleep interruption mothers must cosleep; and on the flipside, cosleeping allows mothers to breastfeed more often, providing more nutrition for a developing infant.

Biologically, our bodies have evolved to both breastfeed and cosleep, and each seems to have helped facilitate the other. So how did this separation occur, and what does it mean for infant well-being and parenting practices in Western societies?

There seem to be distinct reasons for the reduction in breastfeeding and cosleeping in Western societies, yet they obviously affect each other. With respect to breastfeeding, we see the rise of the industrial society, which sent women to work, and science with all its might creating formula, which was believed to be superior to breast milk by doctors for quite some time.

These two factors alone had a huge impact on reducing breastfeeding rates in Western societies. This reduction of breastfeeding meant that sleeping arrangements were also free to change. But in addition, there was an even greater impetus for change—the belief in fostering independence.

Sleep Location and Babies' Independence

The juxtaposition of a baby's dependence/interconnectedness and independence/autonomy has dictated parenting practices around the world, though not always in the same manner. For example, in America the newborn is viewed as entirely dependent upon its mother.

Yet the desired end-goal is for that baby to be an independent and autonomous individual. Thus, our practices are geared towards that end-goal; we put babies alone in their own room, we don't touch them very often, and we've even removed the dependence on mother for breastfeeding through the use of formula.

In contrast, the Japanese view the newborn as an autonomous, independent being who must be held, breastfed, and touched regularly (cosleeping is the norm there), in order to build the feelings of inter-connectedness they value (Caudill & Weinstein, 1969). Similarly, research from New Zealand has found that cultural groups that share the Western-independence view rarely sleep with their infants, while Pacific cultural groups demonstrate lots of sleep contact because they believe that interconnectedness is the way to foster a child's development (Abel, Park, Tipene-Leach, D., Finau, S., & Lennan, M., 2001).

So while there are myriad factors why any one individual would choose to cosleep or not, or breast-feed or not, culturally this notion of independence has played a very large role in shaping our collective views on the issue.

The problem for Western cultures is that the Western assumptions of what fosters independence seem to be, well, wrong. Research has demonstrated that the Eastern interconnectedness model fosters independence and well-being to a much greater degree than simply forcing children to try and be independent.

One such example is the case of the Sami and Norwegian children. Sami individuals are more likely to cosleep with their children, and their children were found to be more independent and demand less attention from their parents than Norwegian children, who typically sleep alone (Arnestad, Andersen, Vege, & Rognum, 2001).

Interestingly, thanks to a push to increase breast-feeding rates in Norway, cosleeping has also become a more common sleeping arrangement (Arnestad et al., 2001), and children are reaping the benefits. Similar relationships have also been found in Sweden, where breastfed infants were much more likely to sleep with their parents than formula-fed infants (Lindgren, Thompson, Haggblom, & Milerad, 1998).

The Logistical Benefits of Bedsharing

I have mentioned some of the logistical reasons for breastfeeding and cosleeping to go together, but is there more than that? After all, if it's a matter of pure logistics, wouldn't it simply be a matter of whatever works to separate the two? Turns out there are a couple of rather important effects that each practice has on the other. Let's start with the effects of cosleeping on breastfeeding. As previously mentioned, cosleeping rates are greater amongst breastfeeding mothers (Blair & Ball, 2004), and while increasing breastfeeding has increased cosleeping rates (Arnestad et al., 2001; Lindgren et al., 1998), the fact is that cosleeping actually *facilitates* more breastfeeding. If you compare mothers who breastfeed, those who cosleep breastfeed up to twice as much at night over those who do not (McKenna, Mosko, & Richard, 1997; See also Ball, this volume).

Why is this important? Dr. Helen Ball has done research on the effects of sleep location on breastfeeding and come to some interesting (though expected) conclusions. Namely, cosleeping right from the start reduces the chances of having breastfeeding problems. Specifically, Dr. Ball looked at sleep locations for new mothers and their infants, and randomly assigned women to one of three location types—either those that facilitated mother-infant access (i.e., bedsharing or putting the infant in a three-sided crib that was attached to the parent bed, much like an official Co-Sleeper), or those that did not (i.e., a stand-alone bassinette next to the mother's bed).

Bedsharing Increases Nighttime Suckling

Mother-infant dyads that had sleeping arrangements that facilitated mother-infant access showed greater successful suckling than those who were in the stand-alone bassinette group (Ball, 2006a). Upon follow-up with these mothers, Dr. Ball found that these effects of early cosleeping continued at 16 weeks, with twice as many mothers in the unhindered-access groups both breastfeeding, and exclusively breastfeeding (Ball & Klingaman, 2007).

This study does not even consider infants in a separate room, as all three groups were room-sharing. But it was the bedsharing (or three-sided crib) that facilitated breastfeeding. Why does this happen? As previously mentioned, infants who cosleep tend to feed (or at least suckle) for twice the amount of time as non-cosleeping infants (Blair & Ball, 2004).

Stimulation of the nipple is necessary for the production of prolactin, the hormone that allows for milk secretion. Thus the reduction in suckling can lead to deleterious effects on milk production or the maintenance of a mother's milk supply (Neville, Morton,& Umemura, 2001). In short, when mothers get their babies into bed with them right away, they reduce the chances of having low milk production when breastfeeding.

Now, what of the effects of breastfeeding on bedsharing? First, you must remember that the biggest argument against bedsharing has to do with infant deaths. Many people argue that bedsharing increases the risk of death via suffocation or SIDS. While there is no direct evidence that breastfeeding *causes* a reduction in SIDS *for bedsharing babies*, there is ample circumstantial evidence to suggest this is the case.

Bedsharing and Breastfeeding Lowers Risk of SIDS

Most prominently, cross-cultural data shows that cultures in which bedsharing *and* breastfeeding are the norm have substantially lower SIDS rates than cultures in which they are not the norm (Lee, Chan, Davies, Lau, & Yip, 1989; Nelson & Taylor, 2001; Watanabe, Yotsukura, Kadoi, Yashiro, Sakanoue, & Nishida, 1994).

For example, Japan has long been considered the pinnacle of success with respect to SIDS deaths, as their rates are generally half of other industrialized nations, and bedsharing is also the norm there. It is possible that breastfeeding has nothing to do with their lower SIDS rates, except that we know breastfed babies are at a much lower risk for SIDS more generally (Ford, Taylor, Mitchell, Enright, Stewart, Becroft, & Scragg, 1993; Fredrickson, Sorenson, Biddle, 1993; Hoffman, Damus, Hillman, & Krongrad, 1988; Ip, Chung, Raman, Chew, Magula, DeVine, Trikalinos, & Lau, 2007; Mitchell, Taylor, Ford, Stewart, Becroft, Thompson, Scragg, Hassall, Barry, & Allen, 1992).

Breastfeeding in and of itself reduces the risk of SIDS. In a meta-analysis on the relationship between breastfeeding and SIDS, researchers found that while any breastfeeding more than halves the risk of SIDS, exclusive breastfeeding has an ever greater effect (Hauck, Thompson, Tanabe, Moon, & Vennemann, 2011). Furthermore, duration and intensity of breast-feeding have also been found to relate to SIDS levels, with greater duration and intensity leading to a lower risk of SIDS (McKenna & McDade, 2005).

Bedsharing babies breastfeed up to twice as long as non-cosleeping babies. It is, therefore, not unreasonable to assume that the extra breastfeeding during cosleeping further increases protection against SIDS.

Breastfeeding and Bedsharing Can Prevent Infant Failure to Rouse

An additional hypothesis for how breastfeeding may reduce the risk of SIDS for cosleeping infants comes from Dr. James McKenna, who has posited that the arousals from breastfeeding keep the infant from falling into a deeper sleep, which may lead to a "failure to rouse" (Mosko, Richard, & McKenna, 1997). This "failure to rouse" has been discussed as a potential mechanism behind SIDS; infants reach too deep a level of sleep and they are simply incapable of coming out of it, similar to entering a coma.

Breastfeeding, thus, increases the number of infant arousals (though not full wakings), and this is greater during cosleeping, and is especially true for breastfeeding dyads not only because of mother's movements, but because of the frequency of feedings.

Breastfeeding and Infant Sleep Position

Another way in which breastfeeding may help reduce the risk of SIDS is by influencing the position in which the infant sleeps. Breastfeeding infants are less likely to sleep prone because it doesn't facilitate breastfeeding; in order for an infant to breastfeed, he or she needs to be on his or her back or side. An infant in the prone position simply cannot reach or latch onto the breast (unless the prone position is on mother). Infant position also helps reduce the chances of infants suffocating, as a baby in the prone position who cannot roll over, is at greater risk for suffocation.

Breastfeeding Impacts Mothers' Sleep Behaviors

Breastfeeding also seems to be related to practices that reduce the risk for suffocation. Research has found that maternal-infant behavior during sleep is different for mothers who breastfeed compared to mothers who formula-feed (Ball, 2006b). Behaviors, such as facing the infant and having the infant lie at chest level, being much more prominent in breastfeeding dyads. These behaviors may seem trivial, but they can be imperative for keeping an infant safe.

For example, a child who lies at chest level (as opposed to head level, which is what Dr. Ball found to be more common in formula-fed infants who coslept) is less likely to be surrounded by pillows, which increases the risk for suffocation. They are also less likely to be too close to a headboard, which is another known hazard. Babies have fallen between the headboard and mattress, and suffocated.

There is also more eye contact between mother and baby during a breastfeeding session than during a bottle-feeding session (Else-Quest, Hyde, & Clark, 2003). Bonding that occurs during daytime feedings may serve to heighten the mother's awareness of her baby, leading her to be intuitively safer at night. That is, a mother who has bonded with her child is more aware of her child's presence at any given point. This has not been formally studied. But it is plausible that the security of attachment between mother and baby may also protect babies while they sleep.

The Benefits of Bedsharing and Breastfeeding

Hopefully, the link between breastfeeding and cosleeping is now clear. The benefits they offer each other are neither superfluous nor easily available by other means. In changing our parenting practices, we have developed other problems. Western countries have alarmingly high rates of breastfeeding problems, and much higher rates of infant mortality (notably SIDS), than other countries who have similar medical advancements, but also breastfeed and bedshare on a regular basis.

Interestingly, we also have a high rate of sleeplessness by new mothers—so much so that we joke about never sleeping again when people have a new baby—and our children have unusually strong attachments to objects for sleep (e.g., security blankets, stuffed animals). Neither of these is universal. In fact, research has shown that breastfeeding mothers who cosleep get more sleep than both bottle-feeding mothers and mothers who breastfeed, but do not bedshare (Quillin & Glenn, 2003, Kendall-Tackett, Cong, & Hale, 2011).

Additionally, children who are solitary sleepers show a greater need and use for security objects and sleep aids (Hayes, Roberts, & Stowe, 1996). So not only do our sleep and feeding practices have significant consequences (i.e., breastfeeding troubles and infant death), we see smaller consequences in the majority of new mothers and their children. Isn't it time we recognized not only the benefits of bedsharing and breastfeeding, but the symbiotic nature of the two?

References

Abel, S., Park, J., Tipene-Leach, D., Finau, S., & Lenan, M. (2001). Infant care practices in New Zealand: A cross-cultural qualitative study. *Social Science & Medicine, 53,* 1135–1148.

Arnestad, M., Andersen, M., Vege, A., & Rognum, T.O. (2001). Changes in the epidemiological pattern of sudden infant death syndrome in southeast Norway, 1984–1998: Implications for future prevention and research. *Archives of Diseases of Childhood, 85,* 180–185.

Ball, HL. (2006a). Bed-sharing on the post-natal ward: Breastfeeding and infant sleep safety. *Journal of the Canadian Paediatric Society, 11,* 43A–46A.

Ball, H.L. (2006b). Parent-infant bed-sharing behavior: Effects of feeding type, and presence of father.*Human Nature, 17,* 301–316.

Ball, H.L., Blair, P.S., & Ward-Platt, M.P. (2004). "New" practice of bedsharing and risk of SIDS. *The Lancet, 363,* 1558.

Ball, H.L., & Klingaman, K.P. (2007). Breastfeeding and mother-infant sleep proximity: Implications for infant care. In: W. Trevathan, E.O. Smith EO, & J.J. McKenna (Eds.) *Evolutionary medicine, 2nd Ed* (226-241). New York: Oxford University Press.

Blair, P.S., & Ball, H.L. (2004). The prevalence and characteristics associated with parent-infant bed-sharing in England. *Archives of Diseases of Childhood, 89,* 1106-1110.

Caudill, W., & Weinstein, H. (1969). Maternal care and infant behaviour in Japan and America. *Psychiatry, 32,* 12–43.

Duijts, L., Jaddoe, V.W.V., Hofman, A., & Moll, H.A. (2010). Prolonged and exclusive breastfeeding reduces the risk of infectious diseases in infancy. *Pediatrics, 126,* e18-e25.

Else-Quest, N.M., Hyde, J.S., & Clark, R. (2003). Breastfeeding, bonding, and the mother-infant relationship. *Merrill-Palmer Quarterly, 49*, 495-517.

Ford, R.P., Taylor, B.J., Mitchell, E.A., Enright, H.W., Stewart, A.W., Becroft, D.M., & Scragg, R. (1993). Breastfeeding and the risk of sudden infant death syndrome. *International Journal of Epidemiology, 22*, 885–890.

Fredrickson, D.D., Sorenson, J.F., & Biddle, A.K. (1993). Relationship of sudden infant death syndrome to breast-feeding duration and intensity. *American Journal of Diseases of Children, 147*, 460.

Hauck, F.R., Thompson, J.M.D., Tanabe, K.O., Moon, R.Y., & Vennemann, M.M. (2011). Breastfeeding and risk of sudden infant death syndrome: A meta-analysis. *Pediatrics, 128*, 1-10.

Hayes, M.J., Roberts, S.M., & Stowe, R. (1996). Early childhood co-sleeping: Parent-child and parent-infant nighttime interactions. *Infant Mental Health Journal, 17*, 348-357.

Hoffman, H., Damus, K., Hillman, L., & Krongrad, E. (1988). Risk factors for SIDS: Results of the institutes of child health and human development SIDS cooperative epidemiological study. In P. Schwartz, D. Southall, & M. Valdes-Dapena (Eds.), *Sudden infant death syndrome: Cardiac and respiratory mechanisms* (Annals of the New York Academy of Science). New York: National Academy of Sciences.

Ip, S., Chung, M., Raman, G., Chew, P., Magula, N., DeVine, D., Trikalinos, T., & Lau, J. (2007). *Breastfeeding and maternal and infant health outcomes in developed countries.* Evidence report/technology assessment number 153. Agency for Healthcare Research and Quality, Rockville, MD (2007). http://www.ahrq.gov/clinic/tp/brfouttp.htm

Lee, N.Y., Chan, Y.F., Davies, D.P., Lau, E., & Yip, D.C.P. (1989). Sudden infant death syndrome in Hong Kong: Confirmation of low incidence. *British Medical Journal, 298,* 721.

Lindgren, C., Thompson, J.M.D., Haggblom, L., & Milerad, J. (1998). Sleeping position, breastfeeding, bedsharing and passive smoking in 3-month-old Swedish infants. *Acta Paediatrica, 87,* 1028–1032.

McKenna, J.J., Ball, H.L., & Gettler, L.T. (2007). Mother-infant co-sleeping, breastfeeding and sudden infant death syndrome: What biological anthropology has discovered about normal infant sleep and pediatric sleep medicine. *Yearbook of Physical Anthropology, 50,* 133-161.

McKenna, J.J., & McDade, T. (2005). Why babies should never sleep alone: A review of the co-sleeping controversy in relation to SIDS, bedsharing and breast feeding. *Paediatric Respiratory Reviews, 6,* 134-152.

McKenna, J.J., Mosko, S., & Richard, C. (1997). Bedsharing promotes breast feeding. *Pediatrics, 100,* 214–219.

Mitchell, E.A., Taylor, B.J., Ford, R.P.K., Stewart, A.W., Becroft, D.M., Thompson, J.W., Scragg, R., Hassall, I.B., Barry, D.M., & Allen, E.M. (1992). Four modifiable and other major risk factors for cot death: The New Zealand study. *Journal of Paediatric & Child Health, Suppl 1,* S3–S8.

Mosko, S., Richard, C., & McKenna, J.J. (1997). Infant arousals during mother-infant bed sharing: Implications for infant sleep and sudden infant death syndrome research. *Pediatrics, 100,* 841-849.

Nelson, E.A.S., & Taylor, B.J. (2001). International child care practices study: Infant sleeping environment. *Early Human Development, 62,* 43–55.

Neville, M.C., Morton, J., & Umemura, S. (2001). Lactogenesis: The transition from pregnancy to lactation. *Pediatric Clinics of North America, 48,* 35-52.

Quillin, S.I.M., & Glenn, L.L. (2003). Interaction between feeding method and co-sleeping on maternal-newborn sleep. *Journal of Gynecology and Neonatal Nursing, 33,* 580-588.

Uvnas-Moberg, K. (2003). *The oxytocin factor: Tapping the hormone of calm, love, and healing.* Cambridge, MA: Da Capo Press.

Watanabe, N., Yotsukura, M., Kado,i N., Yashiro, K., Sakanoue, M., & Nishida, H. (1994). Epidemiology of sudden infant death syndrome in Japan. *Acta Paediatrica Japan, 36,* 329–332.

Reprinted from Evolutionary Parenting, http://evolutionaryparenting.com/we-go-together-like-breastfeeding-and-co-sleeping/, posted July 19, 2011. Used with permission.

5

Who Sleeps with Their Baby and Why?

Helen Ball

More babies bedshare in the first few weeks of life than at any other age. On any given night between 20% and 25% of babies under 3 months of age spend some time sharing a bed with a parent, and during their first three months up to 70% of babies in Euro-American households will have bedshared once or more (Ball, 2009; Blair & Ball, 2004; McCoy, Hunt, Lesko, Vezina, Corwin, Willinger, Hoffman, & Mitchell, 2004). When parents are interviewed about sleeping with their baby they give various reasons for doing so (Ateah & Hamelin, 2008; Ball, 2003; Culver, 2009).

Their answers express deeply rooted cultural or religious beliefs and parenting philosophies, invoke the physiological links between lactation and nighttime breastfeeding, and reflect the biological compulsion that drives bonding and the urge for close contact. On a practical level they also explain that sleeping with the baby makes nighttime care easier, helps them to monitor the baby, provide comfort, and yet obtain sleep.

Other parents report having nowhere else to put their baby at night, or that they have fallen asleep with their baby unintentionally. For breastfeeding mothers all of these reasons may apply, and so it is unsurprising that the largest group of bedsharers, around the globe, are breastfeeding mothers. Although it is a well-established fact that the majority of breastfeeding mothers sleep with their babies, the frequency and patterning with which they do so varies. Some do it all night, every night; some for part of the night; some only occasionally; and some accidentally fall asleep while feeding without ever meaning to.

Although many breastfeeding mothers report having been told that bedsharing is "wrong," almost every breastfeeding mother sometimes falls asleep with her baby, in bed or in a chair, or on a couch, regardless of whether or not she considers herself to be a "bedsharer." The "wrongness" of bedsharing may refer to a caution that it is unsafe—bearing the implication that to bedshare is irresponsible—or "wrong" may express a value judgment that parent-infant bedsharing is morally or culturally inappropriate.

However expressed or interpreted, the labeling of bedsharing as "wrong" is intended to invoke fear or guilt in the parent. It is vital, therefore, that all health professionals who support breastfeeding mothers are well informed about the issues surrounding sleep-sharing, and can help new mothers to make sense of how the research evidence relates to their own situations.

Questions, Questions, Questions...

Of course, many questions surround parent-infant sleep-sharing (be it in an adult bed, or sleeping together elsewhere). Does it "cause" SIDS (cot death)? Does it protect babies from SIDS? Do babies get smothered or overlain? Do mothers get more sleep, or less sleep? Is it dangerous to sleep with your baby if you don't breastfeed? What about babies who are very young, or premature, or very small? What if the parents smoke or drink? Does sleep-sharing help mothers to breastfeed? Does breastfeeding protect babies from sleepsharing risks? Where should you feed at night? Is it better to feed sitting up at night or lying down? How do you bedshare? Can you make the bed safe?

The issues surrounding bedsharing are not simple, and so many of the questions posed do not have simple answers. The research evidence is contradictory, and so is the guidance issued by different organizations. Most of the questions are also not easy to research, because bedsharing is difficult to disentangle from many other aspects of parenting that contribute to various outcomes, and very little research into bedsharing risks considers breastfed and non-breastfed infants separately.

What we know, therefore, is incomplete, and guidance comes with a certain "spin" that reflects the remit or priorities of the organization providing the guidance (Ball & Volpe, 2012) Parents therefore have to use their judgment in determining what works, or is "best," or is "safest," for them and their baby—and they need information in order to do so.

Over the past year, my colleague, Dr. Charlotte Russell, and I have been working with several organizations in the UK (La Leche League, National Childbirth Trust, UNICEF Baby-Friendly Initiative) to produce an Infant Sleep Information website (ISIS) that aims to inform parents and health care providers about the research evidence available on where and how babies sleep (www.isisonline.org.uk). This editorial will summarize some of the issues we discuss on the site, and consider how the latest research is informing parents and health care providers.

Why is Bedsharing Considered Dangerous?

There is a long history to the discussion of infant sleep and safety that begins in our evolutionary past. When I talk to public audiences, I often explain the evolutionary characteristics of human infants and why human mothers and infants require close physical contact with one another in the first few months of life. Because human babies are not completely developed at birth, they need to be closely protected for several weeks, need to be fed often, including at night.

My intention is to explain why mothers often feel a need to sleep with their babies, and why babies respond positively to close contact. Although this sleep contact is a part of our evolved biology, it does not mean it is without risk. I sometimes see biological explanations used as an argument to dismiss safety concerns (e.g., "other mammals sleep with their babies without hurting them").

While it is absolutely the norm among mammals for mothers and their offspring to sleep in close contact, we should remember that it is also common in nature for mammals to die in infancy. Likewise infant mortality has occurred at a high rate throughout human history and babies have died while sleeping with their mothers, for reasons that could be accidental, deliberate, or unrelated to where the baby slept. One aspect of infant mortality that came under early scrutiny was death due to overlying, which in the European Middle Ages was considered to be covert infanticide (Spinelli, 2003), and then in 19th century Scotland was linked to maternal alcohol consumption (Russell-Jones, 1985). To eliminate deliberate or accidental overlying deaths, the *Arcuccio* was invented in Italy to protect infants from their sleeping mothers (National Library of Medicine, 1895) (Figure 1).

Figure 1

The *Arcuccio*

An apparatus to prevent the overlying of infants. *British Medical Journal,* August 10, 1895. In other countries devices long used for infant carrying and daytime infant sleep (e.g., cradles and baskets) became co-opted as nighttime infant sleep spaces as, with increasing prosperity, houses expanded and private bedrooms became fashionable. These influences have resulted in culturally derived infant-sleep practices in many post-industrial nations that are now out of step with mother-infant evolved biology. This discordance between the recent cultural history, and the evolved history of infant care, is at the root of the bedsharing issue.

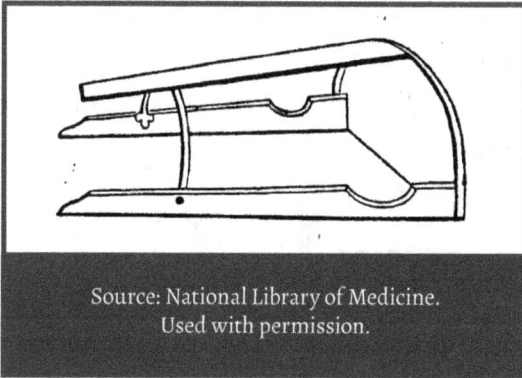

Source: National Library of Medicine.
Used with permission.

As living standards and hygiene improved in prosperous countries during the 19th and 20th centuries, infant death rates declined to what are now their lowest points ever. One goal of Western medicine–to eliminate all preventable infant death—has been pursued extremely successfully in such settings, and as medical knowledge advanced, doctors with incubators and artificial feeding methods at their disposal could keep babies alive without a mother.

Eventually, mothers became superfluous to their infants' survival. By the mid-20th century Western infants predominantly slept in their own room, in specially designed furniture, and were fed chemically modified cow's milk formula. But although the presumed dangers of mothers' sleeping bodies were now absent, inexplicably, babies still died in their cribs, a phenomenon that became colloquially known as cot or crib death. Today Child Death Review Panels,

Infant Mortality Boards, and Safeguarding Committees are prominent in many countries, and stringently examine every infant and child death in pursuit of future prevention.

Introducing SIDS ...

From 1965 the unexpected death of an infant for which no cause could be found at post-mortem was classified as Sudden Infant Death Syndrome (SIDS), with a new code incorporated into the International Classification of Disease. SIDS, therefore, is not a cause from which babies die, but a category to which they are assigned if no cause can be found for their death. The search for the mechanisms underlying these deaths has so far been unsuccessful; it is still not known why babies die unexpectedly in their sleep. However, certain circumstances have been found to be associated with SIDS, such as prone sleep position, exposure to smoking, and lack of breastfeeding.

These circumstances are commonly known as risk factors, and when multiple risk factors affect a single infant the risk of SIDS dramatically increases. Some risk factors are associated with intrinsic infant vulnerability, such as premature birth, low birthweight, or prenatal smoke exposure. Once a baby has been born, these factors cannot be altered. However, other factors are related to the environment of infant care, and are thought to provide a stressor that a vulnerable baby experiencing a critical period of development may be unable to overcome, the so-called "triple-risk SIDS model" (Filiano & Kinney, 1994).

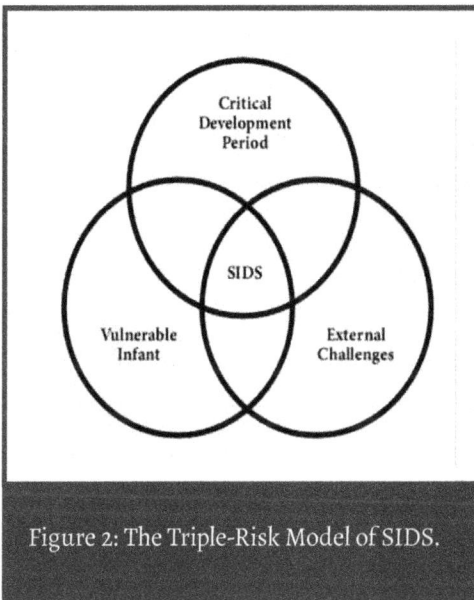

Figure 2: The Triple-Risk Model of SIDS.

These aspects of infant care are generally considered to be "modifiable" risks (e.g., sleep position, overwrapping, head-covering, feeding, pacifier use, parental smoking), and form the basis of many national SIDS prevention campaigns. A large measure of success has been achieved with some simple campaigns (such as "Back to Sleep"), but such "magic bullets" are rare and may actually now be hindering further SIDS-reduction efforts (Ball & Volpe, 2012).

... And Bedsharing

In 1986, anthropologist James McKenna hypothesized that one explanation for SIDS may involve the separation of babies from their mothers at night, a feature of infant care in certain Western countries that is historically and cross-culturally unique (McKenna, 1986). SIDS research at the time implicated suppressed infant arousals and breathing pauses (central apnea) as potential precursors to unexpected infant deaths, and McKenna proposed that infants sleeping in the sensory-rich environment of close sleep contact may be protected from apneic pauses and lack of arousal by maternal sounds, movements, and breathing (McKenna, Mosko, Dungy, & McAninch, 1990).

This was a popular hypothesis that many parents embraced, particularly those who already valued sleep contact with babies for the philosophical or practical reasons mentioned above. Although McKenna's research demonstrated the existence of a high degree of physiological synchrony between sleeping mothers and babies (McKenna, Ball, & Gettler, 2007), research on shared sleep environments indicated that bedsharing was another factor associated with increasing rather than decreasing risk of SIDS, and that the combination of bedsharing with a parent who smokes was particularly implicated (Blair, Fleming, Smith, Mitchell, & Scragg, 1993).

For the past 20 years, discussion and studies regarding the real and presumed risks and benefits of bedsharing have been on-going. No epidemiological studies have produced evidence that bedsharing definitely reduces SIDS risk, although there is strong evidence that co-sleeping (baby room-sharing with parent(s) for sleep) is protective. It is also now clear that certain behaviors and environments interact to make some forms of adult-infant sleep-sharing particularly hazardous (Blair, Fleming, Smith, Platt, Young, Nadin, Berry, & Golding, 1999; Mitchell & Scragg, 1993).

What Are the Risks?

Studies on the association between bedsharing and SIDS have been contradictory, with some finding evidence of an increased risk between bedsharing and SIDS only for the infants of smokers, and others finding the same association for non-smokers also. This has led to some countries and organizations advising parents to never bedshare, and others to avoid bedsharing under certain circumstances. The research evidence was recently reviewed in a meta-analysis that examined the data from 11 national case-control studies with data on SIDS and sleep location conducted between 1987 and 2006 (Vennemann, Hense, Bajanowski, Blair, Complojer, Moon, & Kiechl-Kohlendorfer, 2012).

Three studies were from the U.S., four from the UK, one each from Germany, Ireland, New Zealand and Norway. The review used a broad definition of bedsharing that encompassed the sharing of any sleep surface between adults and young children. Overall, the risk for SIDS increased almost three times for bedsharing in any sleep surface. Maternal smoking data were only available from four studies producing a six-fold increase in risk for maternal smoking and bedsharing (any sleep surface), compared to a 1.66 increase for non-smoking mothers, indicating a significantly increased risk only for smokers. Data on infant age and bedsharing (any sleep surface) were available from just three studies and were examined for all cases, regardless of smoking status.

The risk for infants less than 12 weeks old was about 10 times higher than for infants 12 weeks and older. However, without a further breakdown by smoking status, and no information on the type of sleep surface (e.g., bed vs. sofa), this apparent increased risk for younger infants is difficult to contextualize. It should also be remembered that the 12-week age-bracket is an arbitrary cut-off point and the definition of a "young infant" varies from study to study. In two studies routine bedsharing (any sleep surface) was not associated with SIDS, but five studies revealed a SIDS increase of over two-fold when sleep-sharing was not part of routine practice. Although described as a meta-analysis of 11 studies, only the overall risk of SIDS in relation to "bedsharing" actually incorporates data from the full-range of studies examined.

Where subgroup analyses were undertaken, these involved data from fewer than half the studies at best, and variables were examined in isolation from one another. It is frustrating to not have clear information on whether smoking status, or non-routine sleep-sharing, presents a disproportionately greater risk for young infants or what the contribution of sofa-sharing or alcohol consumption might be in this apparently vulnerable age group.

While this recent meta-analysis predominantly reviewed data that are now fairly old (including data from before and during the Back-to-Sleep campaigns, and the dramatic fall in SIDS deaths during the 1990s), more recent studies provide further insights. Where SIDS prevention guidance has emphasized cot/crib safety (supine sleep, avoidance of head covering and over-wrapping, removal of duvets, soft toys and bumpers, etc.) the rate of SIDS occurring in cots has fallen. Researchers are now beginning to apply the same principles to identifying factors involved in bedsharing safety.

Sleep location was examined in England by SWISS (South West Infant Sleep Study), a four-year population-based case-control study that compared 80 infant deaths meeting the criteria for SIDS with data from two age-matched control groups. The term "cosleeping" was used to define any sleep-sharing between an adult and baby on a bed or a sofa (Blair, Sidebotham, Evason-Coombe, Edmonds, Heckstall-Smith, & Fleming, 2009).

Among the SIDS infants, 54% died while co-sleeping compared with 20% who shared the reference sleep in both control groups. A significant interaction was found for infant deaths between co-sleeping and recent parental use of alcohol or drugs (31% vs. 3% random controls), and co-sleeping on a sofa (17% vs. 1%). The authors concluded that many of the SIDS infants had slept with an adult in a hazardous environment. The major influences on risk, regardless of markers for socioeconomic deprivation, were the use of alcohol or drugs before sharing a bed, and sofa-sharing.

Although data on whether or not mothers "attempted to breastfeed" were compared for cases and controls, no association was found with SIDS.

However, more specific data on infant feeding type at time of death or reference sleep were not reported. It is now clear which characteristics of the shared sleep environment increase the risk of SIDS–smoking, alcohol and drug use, and sleeping with a baby on a sofa–and often these occur in combination. A study of bedsharing infant deaths in Alaska, for instance, found that in 99% of cases, at least one risk factor was present (e.g., maternal tobacco use; sleeping with a person impaired by consumption of some substance affecting awareness or arousal), and concluded that bedsharing alone does not increase the risk of infant deaths (Blabey & Gessner, 2009).

What about Accidental Infant Deaths, Such as Suffocation and Overlying?

In addition to SIDS that may occur during bedsharing, there is a growing literature on sleep location and accidental sudden unexpected death in infancy (SUDI). Distinguishing between SIDS and accidental SUDI has always been difficult due to the absence of clear diagnostic criteria for separating SIDS and soft suffocation. Where evidence for potential suffocation is circumstantial (e.g., presence of a sleep-partner), coroners may designate an infant death as "unascertained." Shared sleep environments have been implicated in infant suffocation deaths in recent UK and U.S. studies (Schnitzer, Covington, & Dykstra, 2012; Weber, Risdon, Ashworth, Malone, & Sebire, 2012).

Therefore, in addition to the issue of whether bedsharing carries an increased SIDS-risk in a given context, all parents should be alert to the possibility of accidental infant deaths when sleep-sharing. Parental responsibility is an important issue for both SIDS and accidental SUDI. If parents have considered safety issues related to bedsharing in advance of sleeping with their baby for the first time, the risks of accidentally falling asleep with the baby in a hazardous environment can be modulated. This is particularly important when alcohol and/or other drugs temporarily impair parental judgment, since it is a sober adult that should be making the decision about a baby's safety.

Breastfeeding and Bedsharing: What Do We Know?

Research confirms what breastfeeding mothers often report: that bedsharing facilitates frequent nighttime breastfeeding. Various studies have found that although bed-sharing breastfeeding mothers wake frequently to feed, they also wake for shorter periods, fall back to sleep more rapidly (Mosko, Richard, &

McKenna, 1997), and achieve greater sleep duration (Quillan & Glenn, 2004), when compared to not bedsharing.

Recently a Swedish study reported an association between bedsharing and three or more nighttime wakings, but interpreted this as an association with sleep problems rather than as the need of breastfed infants to feed frequently, including at night (Mollborg, Wennergren, Norvenius, & Alm, 2011). Although the same authors reported an association in Sweden between bedsharing and being a single parent, in the UK we found the opposite association, with fewer single mothers bedsharing than those who were cohabiting (Ball, Moya, Fairley, Westman, Oddie, & Wright, 2012). Other studies have determined that breastfeeding is associated with greater or equivalent sleep duration than formula-feeding in general, but have not examined sleep location (Doan, Gardiner, Gay, & Lee, 2007; Montgomery-Down, Clawges, & Santy, 2010).

The close interaction between breastfeeding and bedsharing has now been documented in 20 or more studies. Of particular interest is the observed association between bedsharing and greater duration of breastfeeding. In Brazil, for instance, researchers investigated breastfeeding outcomes at 12 months by interviewing mothers of 4,231 infants at birth, 3 and

12 months about their breastfeeding and bedsharing characteristics (Santos, Mota, Matijasevich, Barros, & Barros, 2009). Bedsharing was defined as habitual sharing of a bed between mother and child for all or part of the night. Breastfeeding prevalence at 12 months was 59% for those who bedshared at 3 months, and 44% for those who did not.

Among infants exclusively breastfed at 3 months, 75% of bedsharers were still breastfed at 12 months, versus 52% of non-sharers. The authors accepted these results as evidence that bedsharing protected against early weaning. However, the association tells us nothing about the direction of causality. The relationship may simply be that mothers who are inclined to breastfeed for longer may also be more inclined to bedshare.

Several years ago, we found a significant difference in breastfeeding frequency and infant sleep location when we conducted a randomized video study on the first two nights following birth in a hospital postpartum unit (Ball, Ward-Platt, Heslop, Leech, & Brown, 2006). Babies who shared their mothers' bed, or slept in a side-car crib attached to the bed, fed more than twice as frequently as babies who slept in a standard bassinette by the mothers' bed.

Video footage indicated that when babies woke during the night and began rooting for the breast, mothers in close proximity were alert to their feeding cues, and responded promptly. However, mothers whose babies were in a bassinette at their bedside did not feel their infants' movements or respond to their cues. These babies therefore missed many opportunities to initiate and practice latching and suckling, while the mothers did not receive the frequent nipple stimulation and prolactin surges that trigger prompt and copious milk production.

In a subsequent trial, we hypothesized that as sleep contact between mother and baby had been found to increase breastfeeding frequency, and because frequent breastfeeding is known to promote effective lactation, mothers and babies who were encouraged to sleep in close proximity following delivery may experience a longer duration of breastfeeding than those who slept apart, but in the same room (Ball, Ward-Platt, Howel, & Russell, 2011). In this trial, we randomized mothers and newborn infants to two different sleep conditions during their postpartum hospital stay: 1,204 pregnant women with an intention to breastfeed were recruited at a large UK hospital. Half were randomly allocated to normal rooming-in (stand-alone cot at bedside); the other half were allocated to close-contact (side-car crib clamped to the mother's bed-frame).

Following hospital discharge mothers reported weekly on their breastfeeding status and infant at-home sleep location; 870 mothers provided data for up to 6 months. Adjusting for maternal age, education, delivery type, and previous breastfeeding, we found no significant difference between the groups for duration of any or exclusive breastfeeding. Although we did not find that postnatal sleep proximity affected long-term breastfeeding outcomes in a busy tertiary hospital setting, the follow-up data reinforced the findings of previous studies.

Bedsharing at home was common (reported by 67% of side-car recipients vs. 64% of those rooming-in during postnatal stay), and those who bedshared in the first 13 weeks were twice as likely as non-sharers to breastfeed to 6 months (unpublished data). The short duration of current UK postpartum hospitalization means the directionality of the association now needs examining in the home, but how to randomize mothers and infants to different sleep locations (and ensure compliance) in a domestic setting is a methodological problem still to be solved!

Overall, to date we know that when new breastfeeding mothers bedshare they are more aware of and responsive to their infants' feeding cues, which assists with breastfeeding initiation. In the weeks and months following birth, breastfeeding mothers commonly bedshare to make nighttime feeding easier to manage, and those who bedshare sleep more and breastfeed for longer than those who sleep apart. This may be an important suggestion for working mothers who continue to breastfeed once they return to work, or decide to stop breastfeeding because they are soon returning to work. Even if they wake more often during the night to breastfeed their infants, in general they sleep as many hours or more than non-cosleepers (an advantage for themselves), and they continue to breastfeed for an overall longer period (an advantage for their baby).

Now we must consider the degree to which the benefits of bedsharing for breastfeeding mothers and babies are offset by real or presumed risks.

Breastfeeding, Bedsharing, and Risks

Breastfed babies are sometimes the victims of SIDS, although SIDS deaths are less frequent among babies who are breastfed than those who are not. A meta-analysis of breastfeeding and SIDS confirmed that breastfed babies had less than half the risk of SIDS than those who were not breastfed, and that the effect was stronger when breastfeeding was exclusive (Hauck, Thompson, Tanabe, Moon, & Vennemann, 2011). However, no SIDS case-control studies have determined the SIDS risk of bedsharing in an adult bed by currently breastfeeding infants in the absence of the well-established risks (smoking, alcohol use and drug consumption), with the exception of a study in the Netherlands whose results are considered inconclusive because of the small sample, the lack of breakdown by breastfeeding status, and the lack of data on other risk factors (Ruys, de Jonge, Brand, Engelberts, & Semmekrot, 2007). For all these reasons, this study was excluded from the above meta-analysis.

Other researchers have produced estimates in attempts to address the same issue. Carpenter used data from 20 regions in Europe to estimate that the SIDS-rate for breastfed, bedsharing infants would be twice that of breastfed non-bedsharing infants, reflecting an increase from 1 to 2 per 10,000 in the cumulative number of deaths estimated by 6 months of age (Carpenter, Irgen, Blair, England, Fleming, Huber, Jorch, & Schreuder, 2004). The same estimates for non-breastfed infants produced rates of 4/10,000 and 11/10,000 for not bedsharing and bedsharing respectively.

Compared to the UK national SIDS-rate of 1/2,000, both the estimates for breastfed infants, either in or out of the bedsharing environment, are therefore very low, and an excess risk for non-breastfed babies who bedshare is indicated. In an examination of the patterns of bedsharing and breastfeeding over time between birth and 45 months of age for 14,000 families from the ALSPAC (Avon Longitudinal Study of Parents and Children) cohort study (infants born in 1991 and 1992), latent-class analysis (a powerful multivariate statistical method that identifies unobservable subgroups within a population) was used to identify groups of families based on their bedsharing characteristics (Blair, Heron, & Fleming, 2010).

The authors concluded that families most likely to bedshare in the months following birth were also those most likely to breastfeed, and that the characteristics of these families placed them at very low risk of SIDS. Any benefit from preventing bedsharing in this group, therefore, would be very small, and by following such advice, breastfeeding would probably suffer. The authors recommend that risk-reduction messages to prevent SIDS be targeted specifically to unsafe infant care practices; in this way infant mortality prevention would avoid undermining breastfeeding outcomes for those infants already at low risk of unexpected death.

Balancing Information

The challenge of balancing the public health benefits of exclusive breastfeeding to 6 months of age with the safeguarding/infant mortality agenda of preventing all infant deaths will require creative solutions. Breastfeeding cannot protect an infant from risks introduced by hazardous parental behavior, and so guidance that infants are safest sleeping in a crib next to their parents' bed is defensible as a general public health message; but this message must also acknowledge that not all parent-infant bedsharing is inherently dangerous, and that breastfeeding, bedsharing mothers and infants are a particularly low-risk group.

It is, therefore, not defensible to advise, or imply, that bedsharing is lethal and should never be practiced under any circumstances. To do so is also alienating. Recent data from the U.S., where fear-tactics have been implemented in anti-bedsharing campaigns, indicate that simple messages designed to demonize bedsharing are rejected by the parents at whom they are targeted (Ball & Volpe, 2012). In Milwaukee, the infamous butcher's knife and tombstone messages posted on billboards have failed to produce a sustained reduction in infant mortality in the highest-risk groups.

Cultural infant-care traditions, and personal parenting beliefs that incorporate bedsharing as a valued component of parenting, will not respond to campaigns that treat sleep contact as a modifiable risk factor or simple infant-care practice (such as sleep position). In a recent publication, I argue that much bedsharing research has so far failed to recognize the importance of infant sleep location to ethnic and sub-cultural identity (Ball & Volpe, 2012). We include breastfeeding mothers as a particular subcultural group who reject many of the dominant ideologies regarding infant care, particularly mother-infant separation, and we call for more sensitive and targeted information alongside the continued pursuit of detailed research that helps in the development of more nuanced guidance regarding bedsharing. This is the kind of information we aim to make available on the ISIS website. Please let us know how we're doing (www.isisonline.org.uk).

References

Ateah, C.A., & Hamelin, K.J. (2008). Maternal bedsharing practices, experiences, and awareness of risks. *Journal of Obstetric, Gynecologic, & Neonatal Nursing, 37,* 274-281.

Ball, H. (2009) Airway covering during bed-sharing. *Child Care, Health & Development, 35,* 728-737.

Ball, H.L. (2003). Breastfeeding, bed-sharing, and infant sleep. *Birth, 30,* 181-188.

Ball, H.L., Moya, E., Fairley, L., Westman, J., Oddie, S., & Wright, J. (2012). Bed- and sofa-sharing practices in a UK bi-ethnic population. *Pediatrics, 129,* e673-e681.

Ball, H.L., & Volpe, L.E. (2012). Sudden Infant Death Syndrome (SIDS) risk reduction and infant sleep location—Moving the discussion forward. *Social Science & Medicine;* doi:10.1016/j.socscimed.2012.03.025.

Ball, H.L., Ward-Platt, M.P., Heslop, E., Leech, S.J., & Brown, K.A. (2006). Randomized trial of infant sleep location on the postnatal ward. *Archives of Diseases of Childhood, 91,* 1005-1010.

Ball, H.L., Ward-Platt, M.P., Howel, D., & Russell, C. (2011). Randomized trial of sidecar crib use on breastfeeding duration (NECOT). *Archives of Diseases of Childhood, 96,* 630-634.

Blabey, M.H., & Gessner, B.D. (2009). Infant bed-sharing practices and associated risk factors among births and infant deaths in Alaska. *Public Health Rep, 124,* 527-534.

Blair, P.S., & Ball, H.L. (2004). The prevalence and characteristics associated with parent-infant bed-sharing in England. *Archives of Diseases of Childhood, 89,* 1106-1110.

Blair, P.S., Fleming, P.J., Smith, I.J., Platt, M.W., Young, J., Nadin, P., Berry, P.J., & Golding, J. (1999). Babies sleeping with parents: case-control study of factors influencing the risk of sudden infant death syndrome. CESDI SUDI research group. *British Medical Journal, 319,* 1457-1461.

Blair, P.S., Heron, J., & Fleming, P.J. (2010). Relationship between bed sharing and breastfeeding: longitudinal, population-based analysis. *Pediatrics, 126,* e1119-e1126.

Blair, P.S., Sidebotham, P., Evason-Coombe, C., Edmonds, M., Heckstall-Smith, E.M., & Fleming P. (2009). Hazardous cosleeping environments and risk factors amenable to change: case-control study of SIDS in south west England. *British Medical Journal, 339,* b3666.

Carpenter, R.G., Irgens, L.M., Blair, P.S., England, P.D., Fleming, P., Huber, J., Jorch, G., & Schreuder, P. (2004). Sudden unexplained infant death in 20 regions in Europe: Case control study. *Lancet, 363,* 185-191.

Culver, E.D. (2009). Exploring bed-sharing mothers' motives and decision-making for getting through the night intact: A grounded theory. *Journal of Midwifery and Women's Health.* American College of Nurse-Midwives, Silver Spring MD.

Doan, T., Gardiner, A., Gay, C.L., & Lee, K.A. (2007). Breast-feeding increases sleep duration of new parents. *Journal of Perinatal & Neonatal Nursing, 21,* 200-206.

Filiano, J.J., & Kinney, H.C. (1994). A perspective on neuropathologic findings in victims of the sudden infant death syndrome: The triple-risk model. *Biology of the Neonate, 65,* 194-197.

Hauck, F.R., Thompson, J.M., Tanabe, K.O., Moon, R.Y., & Vennemann, M.M. (2011). Breastfeeding and reduced risk of sudden infant death syndrome: A meta-analysis. *Pediatrics, 128,* 103-110.

McCoy, R.C., Hunt, C.E., Lesko, S.M., Vezina, R., Corwin, M.J., Willinger, M., Hoffman, H.J., & Mitchell, A.A. Frequency of bed sharing and its relationship to breastfeeding. (2004). *Journal of Developmental & Behavioral Pediatrics, 25,* 141-149.

McKenna, J.J. (1986). An anthropological perspective on the sudden infant death syndrome (SIDS): The role of parental breathing cues and speech breathing adaptations. *Medical Anthropology, 10,* 992.

McKenna, J.J., Ball, H.L., & Gettler, L.T. (2007). Mother-infant cosleeping, breastfeeding and sudden infant death syndrome: What biological anthropology has discovered about normal infant sleep and pediatric sleep medicine. *American Journal of Physical Anthropology, Suppl. 45,* 133-161.

McKenna, J.J., Mosko, S., Dungy, C., & McAninch, J. (1990). Sleep and arousal patterns of co-sleeping human mother/infant pairs: A preliminary physiological study with implications for the study of sudden infant death syndrome (SIDS). *American Journal of Physical Anthropology, 183,* 331-347.

Mitchell, E.A., & Scragg, R. (1993). Are infants sharing a bed with another person at increased risk of sudden infant death syndrome? *Sleep, 16,* 387-389.

Mollborg, P., Wennergren, G., Norvenius, S.G., & Alm B. (2011). Bed-sharing among six-month-old infants in western Sweden. *Acta Paediatrica, 100,* 226-230.

Montgomery-Downs, H.E., Clawges, H.M., & Santy, E.E. (2010). Infant feeding methods and maternal sleep and daytime functioning. *Pediatrics, 126,* e1562-e1568.

Mosko, S., Richard, C., & McKenna, J. (1997). Maternal sleep and arousals during bedsharing with infants. *Sleep, 20,* 142-150.

National Library of Medicine. (1895). *The Arcuccio.* Retrieved from: http://www.ncbi.nlm.nih.gov/pmc/articles/PMC2508215/pdf/brmedj08781-0040.pdf

Quillin, S.I., & Glenn, L.L. (2004). Interaction between feeding method and co-sleeping on maternal-newborn sleep. *Journal of Obstetric, Gynecologic, & Neonatal Nursing, 33,* 580-588.

Russell-Jones, D.L. (1985). Sudden infant death in history and literature. *Archives of Diseases of Childhood, 60,* 278-281.

Ruys, J.H., de Jonge, G.A., Brand, R., Engelberts, A.C., & Semmekrot, B.A. (2007). Bed-sharing in the first months of life: A risk factor for sudden infant death. *Acta Paediatrica, 96,* 1399-1403.

Schnitzer, P.G., Covington, T.M., & Dykstra, H.K. (2012). Sudden unexpected infant deaths: Sleep environment and circumstances. *American Journal of Public Health, 102,* 1204-1212.

Santos, I.S., Mota, D.M., Matijasevich, A., Barros, A.J., & Barros, F.C. (2009). Bed-sharing at 3 months and breast-feeding at 1 year in southern Brazil. *Journal of Pediatrics, 155,* 505-509.

Spinelli, M.G. (2003). *Infanticide: psychosocial and legal perspectives on mothers who kill.* Arlington, VA: American Psychiatric Publishing.

Vennemann, M.M., Hense, H.W., Bajanowski, T., Blair, P.S., Complojer, C., Moon, R.Y., & Kiechl-Kohlendorfer, U. (2012). Bed sharing and the risk of sudden infant death syndrome: can we resolve the debate? *Journal of Pediatrics, 160,* 44-48.

Weber, M.A., Risdon, R.A., Ashworth, M.T., Malone, M., & Sebire, N.J. (2012). Autopsy findings of co-sleeping-associated sudden unexpected deaths in infancy: relationship between pathological features and asphyxial mode of death. *Journal of Paediatrics & Child Health, 48,* 335-341.

Reprinted from IBFAN Breastfeeding Briefs, No. 53, Sept 2012, www.ibfan.org/breastfeedingbreafs/bb53. pdf. Used with permission.

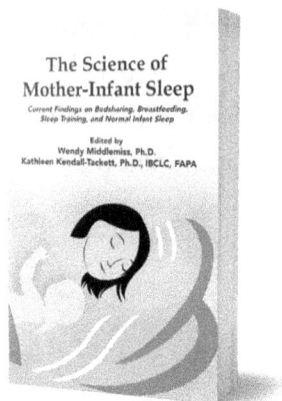

www.ingramcontent.com/pod-product-compliance
Lightning Source LLC
Chambersburg PA
CBHW050535280326
41933CB00011B/1595